Guidelines for Exercise Testing and Prescription

Guidelines for Exercise Testing and Prescription has been written by the Preventive and Rehabilitative Exercise Committee of the American College of Sports Medicine. Many individuals on the committee and others from the College have contributed to each edition. The primary responsibility for writing and editing each edition was assumed by the following editorial committees.

First Edition, 1975:
Karl G. Stoedefalke, Ph.D., Co-Chair
John A. Faulkner, Ph.D., Co-Chair
Samuel M. Fox, M.D.
Henry S. Miller, Jr., M.D.
Bruno Balke, M.D.

Second Edition, 1980:
R. Anne Abbott, Ph.D., Chair
Karl G. Stoedefalke, Ph.D.
N. Blythe Runsdorf, Ph.D.
John A. Faulkner, Ph.D.

Third Edition, 1986:
Steven N. Blair, P.E.D., Chair
Larry W. Gibbons, M.D.
Patricia Painter, Ph.D.
Russell R. Pate, Ph.D.
C. Barr Taylor, M.D.
Josephine Will, M.S.

Fourth Edition, 1991:
Russell R. Pate, Ph.D., Chair
Steven N. Blair, P.E.D.
J. Larry Durstine, Ph.D.
Duane O. Eddy, Ph.D.
Peter Hanson, M.D.
Patricia Painter, Ph.D.
L. Kent Smith, M.D.
Larry A. Wolfe, Ph.D.

Guidelines for Exercise Testing and Prescription

AMERICAN COLLEGE OF SPORTS MEDICINE

4th Edition

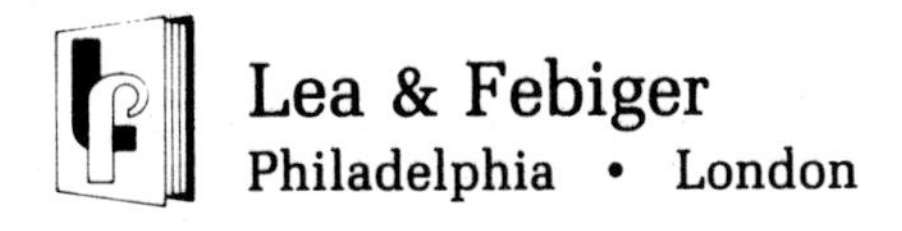

Lea & Febiger
Philadelphia • London

Lea & Febiger
200 Chester Field Parkway
Malvern, Pennsylvania 19355-9725
U.S.A.
(215) 251-2230

Library of Congress Cataloging-in-Publication Data

Guidelines for exercise testing and prescription / American College of Sports Medicine.—4th ed.
p. cm.
Includes bibliographical references.
Includes index.
ISBN 0-8121-1324-1
1. Exercise therapy. 2. Heart—Diseases—Patients—Rehabilitation. 3. Exercise tests. I. American College of Sports Medicine.
[DNLM: 1. Exercise Test. 2. Exercise Therapy. 3. Exertion. WE 103 G946]
RC684.E9G85 1991
615.8′24—dc20
DLC
for Library of Congress

90-13262
CIP

1st Edition, 1975—Reprinted 1976
Reprinted 1977
Reprinted 1979
2nd Edition, 1980—Reprinted 1981
Reprinted 1982 (twice)
Reprinted 1984 (twice)
Reprinted 1985
3rd Edition, 1986—Reprinted 1986
Reprinted 1987 (twice)
Reprinted 1988
Reprinted 1989
Reprinted 1990
4th Edition, 1991

PRINTED IN THE UNITED STATES OF AMERICA

Print number: 9 8 7 6 5 4 3 2

Reprints of chapters may be purchased from Lea & Febiger in quantities of 100 or more.

PREFACE

This fourth edition represents a major step in the evolution of *Guidelines,* a manual first produced by the American College of Sports Medicine in 1975. A volume that began as a concise summary of professional standards for exercise testing and prescription, primarily in cardiac patients, has now become a much more comprehensive document. Standards are now presented for exercise testing and prescription in an entire array of patient populations. Importantly, as much attention is now given to preventive exercise programming in healthy persons as is given to rehabilitative programming for diseased persons.

As compared with the third edition, this edition of *Guidelines* has added new chapters on Clinical Exercise Physiology and Physical Fitness Testing. It is hoped that these additions will enhance the utility of the book, particularly for readers who work in preventive exercise programs and for those who may not have formal training in exercise physiology. Also, major revisions have been made in the chapters on Health Appraisal, Clinical Exercise Testing, Exercise Prescription for Special Populations, Behavior Change, and Administration. These changes have been directed toward incorporating the most current clinical practices and up-to-date, research-based recommendations.

An important modification evident in this edition is a thorough up-dating of the Behavioral Objectives for the various ACSM certifications. These revisions, it is hoped, result in reduced redundancy, greater clarity, and a logical progression of competencies across certification levels. Also, code numbers have been added to facilitate referencing specific behavioral objectives.

One of the most important revisions incorporated into this edition of *Guidelines* is somewhat more subtle than those noted above. Throughout the book, changes have been made that are based on three important observations that have emerged from research over the past decade. Those are: (1) exercise, in moderate amounts and at moderate intensities, is more beneficial to health than previously thought; (2) most adult Americans are either sedentary or participate irregularly in exercise and, therefore, for a large fraction of the population adoption of a regular, moderate exercise program is probably a more realistic goal than is adoption of a vigorous program; and (3) exercise, particularly moderate exercise, is quite safe and consequently expensive medical evaluation is not needed by the vast majority of persons who plan to start a moderate exercise program. These observations have led to recommendations that, it is hoped, have the effect of "sanctioning" participation in a moderate exercise program.

This edition was produced with the assistance of a great many members of the American College of Sports Medicine. The College's gratitude is expressed to all those who contributed ideas, authored sections, reviewed chapters, and provided editorial assistance. In particular, credit is due to all those clinicians and researchers whose efforts continue to expand the body of knowledge concerning exercise testing and prescription.

CONTENTS

CHAPTER 1

Health Appraisal, Risk Assessment, and Safety of Exercise

Sedentary lifestyles are prevalent in industrialized countries. Persuasive evidence now exists to show that regular physical activity protects against the development and progression of several chronic diseases. These two points suggest that considerable public health benefit would result if sedentary persons became more physically active.

A major purpose of this chapter is to state the American College of Sports Medicine's (ACSM) current recommendations regarding appropriate guidelines for health appraisal and risk stratification prior to exercise testing and participation. There is a broad range of opinion on the pertinent issues, and these recommendations represent carefully considered judgments that establish a reasonable compromise between the extreme positions.

RISKS AND BENEFITS OF EXERCISE

It is apparent that there is considerable health benefit associated with quite moderate levels of exercise, although the precise intensity and amount of exercise required for preventing premature morbidity or death is not known specifically. However, it appears that many sedentary individuals would be healthier if they simply took a brisk walk for 30 to 60 minutes every other day.

Although moderate intensity exercise is safe for most individuals, it is desirable for some to have at least a limited health appraisal before starting a vigorous exercise program or performing an exercise test. For many individuals the pre-exercise evaluation can be done by health professionals in nonmedical settings. Age, health status, type of test, and characteristics of the planned exercise are factors that determine the extent of evaluation required and need for medical involvement.

Cardiovascular disease is the leading cause of death in the United States and most of the developed world. Sudden and unexpected death is relatively common in populations with high rates of cardiovascular disease. Most sudden deaths are in middle-aged and older individuals with advanced coronary artery disease (CAD) and occur during a variety of activities, including exercise. It is important to remember that the cause of death in these cases is cardiovascular disease, not exercise, although exercise or a combination of exercise and excitement may be a factor in some instances. Vigorous exercise in persons without underlying cardiovascular disease will not result in sudden death. Death during vigorous exercise is rare, perhaps occurring at the rate of 1 death per year in a population of 15,000 to 20,000 adult exercisers.

Risk of death is transiently increased during the actual exercise period, but is decreased for the rest of the day. The risk of death during exercise must be considered relative to the lower overall death rates seen in physically active groups. The risk of primary cardiac arrest is slightly higher (21 compared to 18 events per 10^8 person-hours) during exercise in regular exercisers than the overall risk for sedentary men.[8] However, the overall risk of cardiac arrest for active men is much lower than sedentary men (5 compared to 18 events per 10^8 person-hours). Other evidence confirms a favorable risk ratio for an active lifestyle. Epidemiological studies consistently show lower all-cause death rates in more physically active groups. In addition, there has been a considerable increase in adult exercise participation over the past 20 years without a concomitant increase in sudden death rates in the United States.

In summary, the risk of serious medical complications during exercise is low, but is higher than during sedentary activities. The overall risk/benefit ratio for an active way of life is favorable. Moderate exercise has the potential to enhance the health of many sedentary individuals and should be widely recommended. Most persons, except for those with known serious disease, can begin a moderate (exercise intensity of 40 to 60% of maximal oxygen uptake [$\dot{V}O_{2max}$]) and gently progressive exercise program, such as walking, without a medical evaluation or exercise test. If there is a question about the safety and suitability of an exercise program for any individual, medical evaluation is recommended.

EXERCISE POLICIES AND SAFETY

Lack of uniformity in guidelines and policies for exercise testing and participation has led to much discussion and concern among exercise program personnel. Issues of primary concern include who should be tested, physician attendance during the test, use of maximal versus submaximal testing, and how to classify individuals into risk groups before and after testing. Previous editions of the *Guidelines* have dealt with these issues, but uncertainty remains.

Some general comments may help put these issues in perspective and help formulate sound policies. There are no guarantees. No matter how rigid and conservative guidelines and policies might be, there is no way to eliminate absolutely the risk of a serious event during exercise testing or exercise participation. Some data are available to estimate the likelihood of an event, but clinical and legal judgment, as well as common sense, must be used to reach judgments on these issues. To cite an extreme example, consider a recommendation that all adults should be given a maximal exercise test with ECG interpretation by a cardiologist prior to starting a walking program. It is conceivable that a few lives might be saved by such a procedure if all sedentary adults in the United States (60 to 70 million persons) were tested, but many people with false positive tests might be discouraged from exercise and thus increase their risk. The recommendation for mass exercise testing is clearly unworkable, and would present such a psychological and economic barrier to exercise participation that fewer persons would be likely to start a program. Many more lives would possibly be lost due to the deleterious effects of sedentary living. However, if no exercise tests were performed, some persons with disease who begin an unsupervised exercise program could potentially have problems. Obviously, a reasonable and prudent approach to exercise testing prior to beginning exercise training that lies between these two extremes must be sought.

A joint report by the American College of Cardiology and the American Heart Association[1] questions the value of diagnostic exercise testing in apparently healthy individuals. The authors of the report state that "exercise testing is of little or no value, inappropriate, or contraindicated" for "asymptomatic, apparently healthy men or women with no risk factors for CAD." The report states that there are no conditions, in the apparently healthy, in which "there is general agreement that exercise testing is justified." The report further states that there are conditions in which "exercise testing is frequently used but . . . there is a divergence of opinion with respect to value and appropriateness." These latter conditions include asymptomatic males in special occupations such as airline pilots, and asymptomatic males over the age of 40 with two or more major risk factors for CAD, or who are sedentary and plan to begin *vigorous* exercise.

The joint report was written from a medical perspective and considered the value of exercise testing for diagnosing disease and patient management. Exercise testing is performed in many situations for nonmedical purposes, such as in worksite health promotion programs, YMCAs and YWCAs, health clubs, and other community exercise programs. This testing is nondiagnostic, in many cases, the ECG is not monitored, and is done to assess physical fitness, to provide a basis for exercise prescription, and to monitor progress in an exercise program. The American College of Sports Medicine believes that this type of nondiagnostic exercise testing is appropriate when conducted with appropriate screening and may be performed by qualified nonmedical testing personnel. Such testing programs may be useful in educating participants about exercise and physical fitness and helping to increase motivation to exercise in sedentary individuals. Fitness testing may have prognostic value beyond the ECG responses to exercise tests. Recent studies show that physically unfit men and women are at higher risk for all-cause and cardiovascular disease mortality.

RISKS OF EXERCISE TESTING

Exercise testing, as currently practiced, is a relatively safe procedure. Recent surveys of more than 2,000 clinical exercise testing laboratories, in which more than 600,000 tests were performed, show a death rate of approximately 0.5 per 10,000 exercise tests. In these surveys, there were different approaches and methods of exercise testing, a variety of populations, and both diagnostic and fitness tests. It is not possible with the currently available data to stratify risk by different populations and methods, but the overall risk as stated above is a reasonable summary estimate. In more than 70,000 maximal exercise tests in one preventive medicine clinic there have been no deaths, and only 6 major medical complications (e.g., myocardial infarction, ventricular fibrillation, dysrhythmias requiring medical treatment, asystole, or stroke). These data suggest that the rate of complications during exercise testing is higher in populations undergoing diagnostic testing, compared to persons being tested as part of a preventive medical examination.

The risks of submaximal physical fitness testing appear to be quite low. The submaximal cycle ergometer test described in Chapter 3 has been administered to approximately 130,000 adults (age 18 to 65 years) over the past decade in several worksite health promotion programs and in community health survey centers. Pretest screening and the exercise testing was performed by nurses or ACSM certified exercise test technologists. There have been no deaths or serious medical complications associated with this submaximal fitness testing. The Canadian Home Fitness Test (currently known as the Canadian Aerobic Fitness Test) has been used around the world over the past 14 years by an estimated 1 million people. No complications more serious than some minor muscle injuries and a few reports of syncope have been reported. Thus, submaximal physical fitness testing appears to have a low risk when accompanied by appropriate pretest screening such as the Physical Activity Readiness Questionnaire (PAR-Q), and can be administered safely by qualified personnel in nonmedical settings.

RISK STRATIFICATION

A careful evaluation of individuals prior to exercise testing or exercise participation is important for numerous reasons including the following: to assure the safety of exercise testing and subsequent exercise programs; to determine the appropriate type of exercise test or exercise program; to identify those in need of more comprehensive medical evaluation; and to make appropriate recommendations for an exercise program. It is recommended that persons interested in participation in organized exercise programs be evaluated by the criteria presented in Tables 1–1 and 1–2. As a minimum standard, the PAR-Q can be used.

Individuals considered for exercise testing or those who plan to increase their physical activity are classified into three risk strata.

1. Apparently healthy—those who are asymptomatic and ap-

Table 1–1. Major Coronary Risk Factors.

1. Diagnosed hypertension or systolic blood pressure ≥ 160 or diastolic blood pressure ≥ 90 mmHg on at least 2 separate occasions, or on antihypertensive medication
2. Serum cholesterol ≥ 6.20 mmol/L (≥ 240 mg/dl)
3. Cigarette smoking
4. Diabetes mellitus*
5. Family history of coronary or other atherosclerotic disease in parents or siblings prior to age 55

*Persons with insulin dependent diabetes mellitus (IDDM) who are over 30 years of age, or have had IDDM for more than 15 years, and persons with non-insulin dependent diabetes mellitus who are over 35 years of age should be classified as patients with disease and treated according to the guidelines in Table 1–3.

Table 1–2. Major Symptoms or Signs Suggestive of Cardiopulmonary or Metabolic Disease.*

1. Pain or discomfort in the chest or surrounding areas that appears to be ischemic in nature
2. Unaccustomed shortness of breath or shortness of breath with mild exertion
3. Dizziness or syncope
4. Orthopnea/paroxysmal nocturnal dyspnea
5. Ankle edema
6. Palpitations or tachycardia
7. Claudication
8. Known heart murmur

*These symptoms must be interpreted in the clinical context in which they appear, since they are not all specific for cardiopulmonary or metabolic disease.

parently healthy with no more than one major coronary risk factor (Table 1–1).

2. Individuals at higher risk—those who have symptoms suggestive of possible cardiopulmonary or metabolic disease (Table 1–2) and/or two or more major coronary risk factors (Table 1–1).
3. Individuals with disease—those with known cardiac, pulmonary, or metabolic disease.

Results of exercise testing may dictate re-classification of individuals prior to exercise training.

RECOMMENDATIONS

No set of guidelines on exercise testing and participation can cover every conceivable situation. Local circumstances and policies vary and specific program procedures are also properly diverse. In an attempt to provide some general guidance on exercise program issues, the American College of Sports Medicine makes the following recommendations (see Table 1–3 for a summary).

APPARENTLY HEALTHY INDIVIDUALS

Apparently healthy individuals can begin **moderate** (intensities of 40 to 60% $\dot{V}O_{2max}$) exercise programs (such as walking or increasing usual daily activities) without the need for exercise testing or medical examination as long as the exercise program begins and proceeds gradually and as long as the individual is alert to the development of unusual signs or symptoms. **Moderate** exercise is further described as being well within the individual's current capacity and can be sustained comfortably for a prolonged period, i.e., 60 minutes. **Vigorous** exercise (intensity $>$ 60% $\dot{V}O_{2max}$) is intense enough to represent a substantial challenge and results in significant increases in heart rate and respiration. **Vigorous** exercise usually cannot be sustained by untrained individuals for more than 15 to 20 minutes. At or above age 40 in men or age 50 in women, it is desirable for individuals to have a medical examination and a maximal exercise test before beginning a **vigorous** exercise program. At any age, the information gathered from an exercise test may be useful to establish an effective and safe exercise prescription. Maximal testing done for men at age 40 or above or women age 50 years and older, even when no symptoms or risk factors are present, should be performed with physician supervision. Submaximal testing up to 75% of age-predicted maximal heart rates in apparently healthy individuals of any age can be done without physician supervision, if the testing is carried out by well-trained individuals (such as ACSM certified personnel) who are experienced in monitoring exercise tests and in handling emergencies.

INDIVIDUALS AT HIGHER RISK

Individuals at higher risk are those with two or more major coronary risk factors (Table 1–1) and/or symptoms suggestive of cardiopulmonary or metabolic disease (Table 1–2). (Metabolic disease includes diabetes mellitus, thyroid disorders, renal disease, liver disease, and other less common diseases of a metabolic type.) An exercise test prior to beginning a vigorous exercise program is desirable for higher risk individuals of any age. For those without symptoms, an exercise test or medical examination may not be necessary if moderate exercise is undertaken gradually with appropriate guidance and no competitive participation. Maximal exercise tests in patients at higher risk should be physician supervised. Submaximal exercise tests

Table 1–3. Guidelines for Exercise Testing and Participation.

	Apparently Healthy		*Higher Risk**		
	Younger ≤ 40 years (men) ≤ 50 years (women)	*Older*	*No symptoms*	*Symptoms*	*With Disease†*
Medical exam and diagnostic exercise test recommended prior to:					
Moderate exercise‡	No§	No	No	Yes	Yes
Vigorous exercise#	No	Yes**	Yes	Yes	Yes
Physician supervision recommended during exercise test:					
Sub-maximal testing	No	No	No	Yes	Yes
Maximal testing	No	Yes	Yes	Yes	Yes

*Persons with two or more risk factors (see Table 1–1) or symptoms (Table 1–2).
†Persons with known cardiac, pulmonary, or metabolic disease.
‡Moderate exercise (exercise intensity 40 to 60% $\dot{V}O_{2max}$)—Exercise intensity well within the individual's current capacity and can be comfortably sustained for a prolonged period of time, i.e., 60 minutes, slow progression, and generally non-competitive.
#Vigorous exercise (exercise intensity > 60% $\dot{V}O_{2max}$)—Exercise intense enough to represent a substantial challenge and which would ordinarily result in fatigue within 20 minutes.
§The "no" responses in this table mean that an item is "not necessary". The "no" response does **not** mean that the item should not be done.
**A "yes" response means that an item is recommended.

are of little diagnostic value in this population, but if such tests are done for non-diagnostic purposes, it is not necessary to have a physician present if the patient is asymptomatic. Persons of any age with symptoms suggestive of coronary, pulmonary, or metabolic disease should have a medical examination and a physician supervised maximal exercise test prior to beginning an exercise program.

PATIENTS WITH DISEASE

A thorough medical evaluation is recommended before starting an exercise program for all individuals with known cardiovascular, pulmonary, or metabolic disease. This is important not only to assess the safety of vigorous exercise, but to measure functional capacity so that progress can be monitored. Diagnostic exercise testing in this group of individuals is valuable in establishing prognosis and making decisions about need for further evaluation or intervention. A physician should be present.

SUMMARY

The health value of regular exercise is confirmed by numerous research studies, and broad recommendations to the public to be physically active are appropriate. There is potential negative impact on physical activity participation from suggesting that exercise is dangerous, or insisting that all sedentary persons receive medical clearance prior to becoming more active. The limited availability of qualified health personnel and facilities in relation to the large volume of medical evaluations and exercise testing required to comply with the recommendations presented in this chapter (Table 1–3) necessitates discretion in their implementation. Most sedentary individuals can begin a moderate exercise program safely; and if large numbers adopt a more active way of life, the public's health will be enhanced. The degree of medical supervision of exercise tests proposed varies appropriately from physician supervised tests to situations in which there may be no physician present. The degree of physician supervision may vary with local policies and circumstances, the health status of the patient, and the experience of the laboratory staff. The appropriate protocol is based on the age, health status, and physical activity level of the person to be tested. All tests should be administered by a person qualified in exercise testing and CPR, preferably a person certified in one of the ACSM certification programs.

REFERENCES

1. American College of Cardiology/American Heart Association: Guidelines for exercise testing. *Circulation 74*:653A–667A, 1986.
2. American Diabetes Association. Exercise and NIDDM. *Diabetes Care 13*:785–789, 1990.
3. Blair SN, Kohl HW, Paffenbarger RS, Clark DG, Cooper KH, and Gibbons LW: Physical fitness and all-cause mortality: A prospective study of healthy men and women. *JAMA 262*:2395–2401, 1989.
4. Ekelund LG, Haskell WL, Johnson JL, Whaley FS, Criqui MH, and Sheps DS: Physical fitness as a predictor of cardiovascular mortality in asymptomatic North American men: The Lipid Research Clinics Mortality Follow-up Study. *N Engl J Med 319*:1379–1384, 1988.
5. Gibbons L, Blair SN, Kohl HW, and Cooper K: The safety of maximal exercise testing. *Circulation 80*:846–852, 1989.
6. Kohl HW et al: Prevalence of abnormal exercise tests by age and health status: An application of the ACSM Guidelines. *Med Sci Sports Exerc,* in press.
7. Shephard RJ: PAR-Q, Canadian Home Fitness Test and exercise screening alternatives. *Sports Med 5*:188–195, 1988.
8. Siscovick DS, Weiss NS, Fletcher RH, and Lasky T: The incidence of primary cardiac arrest during vigorous exercise. *N Engl J Med 311*:874–877, 1984.
9. Thompson PD: The safety of exercise testing and participation. *In* American College of Sports Medicine, *Resource Manual for Guidelines for Exercise Testing and Prescription.* Philadelphia: Lea & Febiger, 1988, pp 273–277.

CHAPTER 2

Clinical Exercise Physiology

A basic understanding of exercise science is essential for health professionals involved in exercise testing and prescription. Of particular importance is knowledge of the physiological systems that function to provide energy for exercise performance. Among these are the oxygen transport system and the metabolic pathways that function in skeletal muscle tissue. This chapter is intended to provide a concise summary of those aspects of exercise physiology that are particularly applicable in the clinical setting.

ENERGY, FORCE, WORK, AND POWER

The ultimate goal of physiological responses to exercise is to provide energy for the performance of physical work. Energy contained in food is converted through the anaerobic and aerobic metabolic pathways described below to form adenosine triphosphate (ATP) and heat. Subsequently, ATP is broken down enzymatically (hydrolyzed) into adenosine diphosphate (ADP) and phosphate (P) to provide energy for muscle contraction and the generation of force (expressed in newtons or kilograms).

$$ATP + H_2O \rightarrow ADP + P + \text{energy}$$

Muscle contraction may be concentric (shortening), eccentric (lengthening), or may involve no movement (static or isometric contraction). If muscle contraction results in mechanical movement, then work has been accomplished (work = force × distance, expressed in joules or kilogram-meters). Power is the rate of performing work, and thus involves a time component [power = force × distance × $time^{-1}$, expressed in watts or kilogram-meters·min^{-1} (kg-m·min^{-1})].

METABOLIC FUNDAMENTALS

Energy for muscular activity is made available by the interaction of three metabolic systems: (1) stored phosphagens, (2) anaerobic glycolysis, and (3) oxidative metabolism. Utilization of these systems depends on the intensity and duration of exercise (see Table 2–1).

ANAEROBIC METABOLISM

An anaerobic process is one that does not require the utilization of oxygen. Energy for muscle contraction can be provided through 2 metabolic pathways that are anaerobic: (1) stored phosphagens and (2) anaerobic glycolysis.

Stored Phosphagens

High intensity, short duration exercise (e.g., 100 m dash) is performed using energy derived primarily from stored phosphagens [ATP and creatine phosphate (CP)]. ATP and CP are high energy compounds that can provide energy for immediate use. ATP is broken down to provide energy and CP donates a phosphate to ADP to reform ATP. This system can be activated quickly and has a high peak power output, but the total capacity for work performance is limited. This is primarily due to the small amounts of stored ATP and CP.

Anaerobic Glycolysis

The second anaerobic pathway, anaerobic glycolysis, is utilized at the beginning of sustained effort prior to the full en-

Table 2–1. Characteristics of the Major Energy Producing Systems.*

System	*Substrate (Fuel)*	*O_2 Required*	*Speed of ATP Mobilization*	*Total ATP Production Capacity*
Anaerobic metabolism				
(a) ATP-CP system	Stored phosphagens	No	Very fast	Very limited
(b) Glycolysis	Glycogen/ glucose	No	Fast	Limited
Aerobic metabolism (TCA cycle, electron transport chain)	Glycogen/ glucose, fats, protein	Yes	Slow	Essentially unlimited

*Adapted from Fox EL and Mathews DK: *The Physiological Basis of Physical Education and Athletics*. Philadelphia: W.B. Saunders, 1981.

gagement of the oxygen transport systems and is also important during sustained high-intensity exercise which requires energy greater than that available from the aerobic processes. Glycolysis involves a series of reactions that degrade glucose to pyruvate or lactate, depending on the availability of oxygen. If sufficient oxygen is available, such as during steady-state exercise, primarily pyruvate is formed. However, if sufficient oxygen is not available to the cells, such as during high intensity exercise, lactate will be formed. The glycolytic system can be activated quickly, but its maximum power and capacity for total work performance are limited.

Some lactate is also formed during rest and sustained submaximal exercise, but does not accumulate because the production and removal rates are equal. The rate of such lactate production is directly proportional to exercise intensity and is related in part to the degree of recruitment of fast-twitch glycolytic (type IIb) muscle fibers.

AEROBIC METABOLISM

The bulk of the energy needed for prolonged physical activity lasting more than approximately 3 minutes is provided by aerobic (i.e., oxidative) metabolism. The aerobic pathways for energy production include the tricarboxylic acid (TCA) cycle (also referred to as Krebs or citric acid cycle) and the electron transport chain. The TCA cycle degrades acetyl CoA (formed from pyruvate or fats) into CO_2 and hydrogen atoms (electrons). The electrons are then shuttled to the electron transport chain for oxidative-phosphorylation and the subsequent regeneration of ATP. The peak metabolic power of the oxidative system is low, but since fat released from adipose tissue is available as a source of energy, the total capacity of this system is substantial. Fatty acid molecules are transformed into acetyl CoA and hydrogen atoms via beta oxidation for entry into the TCA cycle and electron transport chain. The ability to deliver oxygen to contracting skeletal muscle is critical for the performance of prolonged exercise and maximum oxygen uptake ($\dot{V}O_{2max}$) is an important index of the capacity for sustained work performance.

Oxygen uptake ($\dot{V}O_2$) and carbon dioxide production ($\dot{V}CO_2$) during exercise can be determined by open-circuit spirometry. This technique involves measurement of the rate of pulmonary ventilation and analysis of expired air samples for their oxygen and carbon dioxide content. For many practical purposes this is not necessary since the oxygen requirement of performing physical work is known (1 kg·m = 1.8 ml O_2) and is fairly consistent between individuals for the performance of standard exercise tasks. Thus, if the exercise power output is known for activities such as treadmill exercise, cycling and bench stepping, it is possible to estimate the rate of oxygen uptake with reasonable accuracy (Appendix D).

FUEL UTILIZATION

The three fuels available for muscular activity are carbohydrate, fat and protein (Table 2–2). These fuels require different amounts of oxygen to oxidize the molecules to their end products, CO_2 and water. Accordingly, the amount of CO_2 produced in relation to O_2 consumed varies among the three fuels. The ratio of CO_2 produced to O_2 consumed is quantified by the **Respiratory Quotient** (RQ; $\dot{V}CO_2/\dot{V}O_2$). Therefore, RQ can be used to determine which nutrients are being utilized for energy.

When carbohydrate is oxidized completely through the aerobic pathways, the following equation applies:

$$C_6H_{12}O_6 \text{ (glucose)} + 6\ O_2 \rightarrow 6\ CO_2 + 6\ H_2O$$

Note that one mole of carbon dioxide is produced for every mole of oxygen utilized, resulting in a RQ of 1.00.

Fat has a much higher caloric density than carbohydrate (9.3 vs. 4.1 $kcal \cdot g^{-1}$) and is the primary chemical form of stored energy in the body. The following equation describes the oxidation of fat via the citric acid cycle and electron transport chain:

$$2\ C_{51}H_{98}O_6 \text{ (tripalmitin)} + 145\ O_2 \rightarrow 102\ CO_2 + 98\ H_2O$$

Note that more oxygen is required for every mole of CO_2 produced when fat is oxidized, resulting in a RQ of 0.70. Also, slightly less energy is released (4.7 vs. 5.0 $kcal \cdot L^{-1}$) for every

Table 2–2. Substrate Utilization During Exercise.

Fuel	*Energy Content (Kcal · g⁻¹)*	*Oxygen Equivalent (Kcal · L⁻¹)*	*Respiratory Quotient (RQ)*
Carbohydrate	4.1	5.0	1.00
Fat	9.3	4.7	0.70
Protein	4.3	4.4	0.80

liter of oxygen utilized when fat as opposed to carbohydrate is oxidized.

Amino acids can enter the citric acid cycle and can be oxidized to provide energy. Under most circumstances, however, protein utilization during exercise is negligible in terms of energy production and is usually disregarded. The **nonprotein RQ** can be calculated and is often used to describe the gas exchange attributed to the breakdown of only carbohydrates and fats. However, because protein utilization is so low during exercise, RQ and nonprotein RQ are usually similar.

Relative utilization of carbohydrate and fat varies with exercise intensity. During sustained submaximal exercise, a mixture of fat and carbohydrate is used. During prolonged exercise, the percentage of fat utilized also tends to increase gradually over time. As exercise intensity increases, $\dot{V}CO_2/\dot{V}O_2$ rises to reflect greater utilization of carbohydrate and approaches a value of 1.0 near maximal exercise and can exceed 1.0 during heavy nonsteady-state or maximal exercise. This is because the excess CO_2 produced by the body's buffering processes (to compensate for metabolic acidosis) exits through the lungs and is "blown off" under these circumstances. Because this excess CO_2 is being exhaled, the respiratory quotient at the cellular level differs from the lung level. Whereas the RQ describes metabolism as it occurs at the cellular level, the **Respiratory Exchange Ratio** (RER or R) is the $\dot{V}CO_2/\dot{V}O_2$ at the lungs, measured by open circuit spirometry. The calculations for the two values are the same.

MUSCLE PHYSIOLOGY

Human skeletal muscle contains 3 major types of motor units. These include slow twitch oxidative (type I), fast twitch oxidative-glycolytic (type IIa), and fast twitch glycolytic (type IIb) motor units with specific functional characteristics (see Table 2–3).

In general, type I motor units are well-suited for endurance-type activities. Therefore, muscles involved in posture maintenance or prolonged locomotion have a high percentage of type I motor units. Conversely, type II motor units are adapted for strength/power activities and their use results in significant lactate formation. During graded exercise testing, type I units are recruited first with progressively greater involvement of type II units and production of lactate as power output is in-

Table 2–3. Characteristics of Motor Units Comprising Human Skeletal Muscle.

	Type I	*Type IIa*	*Type IIb*
Contraction time	Slow	Fast	Fast
Oxidative capacity	High	Moderate	Low
Myofibrillar ATPase activity	Low	High	High
Stored phosphagens	Low	High	High
Glycolytic capacity	Low	Moderate	High
Fatigability	Low	Low	High

creased. When lactate formation exceeds the maximal rate of removal, lactate accumulates in the blood and leads to muscular fatigue.

MAXIMAL OXYGEN UPTAKE

Maximal oxygen uptake can be measured by open-circuit spirometry, or can be predicted from the peak exercise time or power output achieved during a standard maximal exercise test protocol (e.g., Bruce protocol) or can be predicted from submaximal exercise tests. Values can be expressed either in absolute ($l \cdot min^{-1}$) or weight-relative units ($ml \cdot kg^{-1} \cdot min^{-1}$ or METs). Absolute maximal aerobic power reflects the ability to perform external work. Relative maximal aerobic power is a better reflection of the ability to move one's body and is also related inversely to body fatness. One MET is equivalent to an oxygen uptake of 3.5 $ml \cdot kg^{-1} \cdot min^{-1}$. It is conventional in clinical exercise testing to express $\dot{V}O_{2max}$ in METs (e.g., $\dot{V}O_{2max}$ of 35 $ml \cdot kg^{-1} \cdot min^{-1}$ is equivalent to 10 METs).

From a physiological viewpoint, values for $\dot{V}O_{2max}$ in healthy individuals can be altered by several variables. Within limits, higher values are obtained when a larger muscle mass is involved in testing. Values for incline treadmill running are higher than horizontal treadmill running; running values exceed leg cycle ergometry values; and leg cycle ergometry produces higher values than arm cycle ergometry. In addition, values may be moderately augmented by adding arm exercise to maximal leg exercise. Mean values for women (expressed in $ml \cdot kg^{-1} \cdot min^{-1}$) are approximately 10 to 20% lower than in men of comparable age and physical fitness, primarily due to the higher average body fatness and lower hemoglobin concentration in females. After the age of 25 years, $\dot{V}O_{2max}$ declines approximately 9% per decade. It is unclear how much of this decline is due to the aging process or to reduced physical activity. Finally, $\dot{V}O_{2max}$ is reduced by environmental challenges such as altitude exposure (hypoxia) or air pollution.

DETERMINANTS OF OXYGEN UPTAKE

The ability to take in and utilize oxygen depends on the following physiological processes:

1. Pulmonary ventilation;
2. Diffusion of oxygen from lung alveoli to pulmonary capillary blood;
3. Cardiac performance;
4. Redistribution of blood flow to skeletal muscle vascular beds;
5. Utilization of oxygen and extraction from arterial blood by contracting skeletal muscle.

PULMONARY VENTILATION

Oxygenation of arterial blood depends on alveolar ventilation, gas exchange involving diffusion of oxygen from lung alveoli and pulmonary capillaries and the oxygen carrying capacity of blood. Pulmonary ventilation ($\dot{V}_E$) at $\dot{V}O_{2max}$ reaches a value approximately 20 to 25 times that of the resting state. During moderate exercise, ventilation is increased primarily by increasing tidal volume (V_T), whereas increases in breathing frequency are more important to augment $\dot{V}_E$ during heavy exercise.

At a critical exercise intensity (usually 60 to 70% $\dot{V}O_{2max}$) lactate begins to accumulate in the blood since the rate of production and passage into the bloodstream exceeds the rate of removal by the liver, kidney, and other tissues. This results in reduction in blood pH and an increase in pulmonary ventilation which partly compensates for metabolic acidosis related to lactate accumulation. During a graded exercise test, the power output or rate of oxygen uptake at which ventilation departs from linearity is known as the ventilatory threshold (T_{vent}). Under many circumstances, T_{vent} coincides with the onset of blood lactate accumulation (OBLA) (Fig. 2–1).

Muscular fatigue at an intensity of sustained exercise greater than that of OBLA or T_{vent} is associated with progressive accumulation of lactate in blood. In prolonged exercise at an intensity below OBLA or T_{vent} (e.g., marathon running), blood lactate levels reach a steady state and fatigue is usually asso-

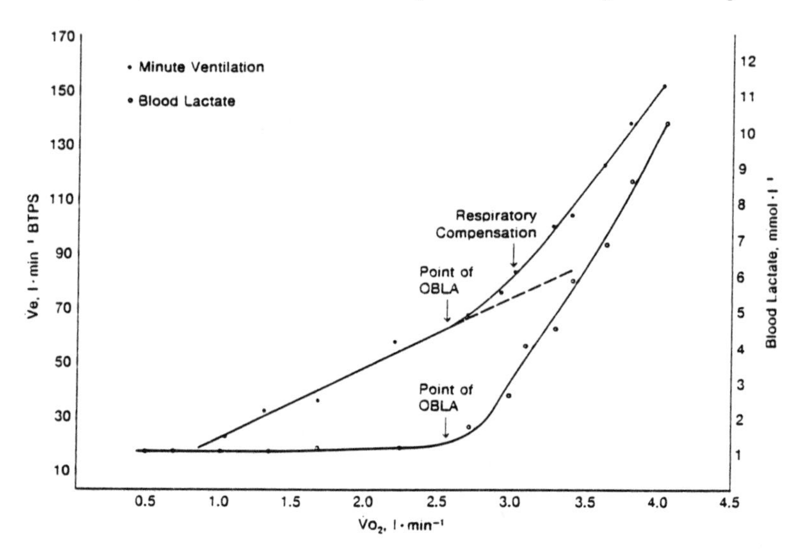

FIGURE 2–1. Pulmonary ventilation, blood lactate, and oxygen consumption during incremental exercise to the maximal oxygen uptake. The dashed line represents the extrapolation of the linear relationship between $\dot{V}_E$ and $\dot{V}O_2$ observed during submaximal exercise. The OBLA is that point at which blood lactate begins to increase above the resting value and is detected by the point at which the relationship between ventilation and oxygen consumption deviates from linearity. "Respiratory Compensation" is a further increase in ventilation to counter the falling pH in anaerobic exercise. Reprinted with permission from McArdle WD, Katch FI, and Katch VL: *Exercise Physiology: Energy, Nutrition, and Human Performance,* 2nd ed. Philadelphia: Lea & Febiger, 1986.

ciated with depletion of muscular glycogen stores. As a result of these relationships, OBLA/T_{vent} is considered by some authorities to be the best available index of the capacity for prolonged exercise. OBLA/T_{vent} can be increased by aerobic conditioning both in absolute ($\dot{V}O_2$, 1·min^{-1} at OBLA) or relative terms (% $\dot{V}O_{2max}$ at OBLA).

GAS EXCHANGE

The process of pulmonary gas exchange depends on the difference in the partial pressure of oxygen (PO_2) between lung alveoli and pulmonary capillary blood and on matching of alveolar ventilation to alveolar perfusion. During exercise, the partial pressure of alveolar oxygen (P_AO_2) rises due to increased alveolar ventilation. The PO_2 of mixed venous blood is also reduced due to greater oxygen uptake by skeletal muscle, resulting in a greater partial pressure gradient for oxygen across the alveolar-capillary membrane. As a consequence of the greater overall alveolar ventilation and opening of pulmonary capillaries, matching of pulmonary ventilation to perfusion is also optimized during exercise. Therefore, the saturation of hemoglobin in arterial blood remains approximately 95% up to maximal exercise in healthy subjects. The oxygen content of arterial blood depends not only on the PO_2 gradient between the lung and the pulmonary capillaries, but also on oxygen carrying capacity of blood. If hemoglobin levels are reduced, the oxygen content of arterial blood will be lowered and $\dot{V}O_{2max}$ may be reduced.

CARDIAC PERFORMANCE

Heart Rate

Intrinsic heart rate, as dictated by spontaneous depolarization of the sinoatrial (SA) node, is approximately 90 beats·min^{-1}. In the resting state, heart rate is reduced to approximately 70 beats·min^{-1} as a result of parasympathetic tone. Heart rate increases during graded exercise first by withdrawal of parasympathetic tone and then by augmentation of sympathetic neural input to the SA node. In healthy individuals, heart rate rises in a linear fashion as a function of increasing oxygen uptake and attains a plateau just prior to achievement of $\dot{V}O_{2max}$ during graded exercise testing (Fig. 2–2). Maximal heart rate is reduced with increasing age. Average values can be *predicted* from the following equation:

$$\text{Predicted maximal heart rate} = 220 - \text{age.}$$

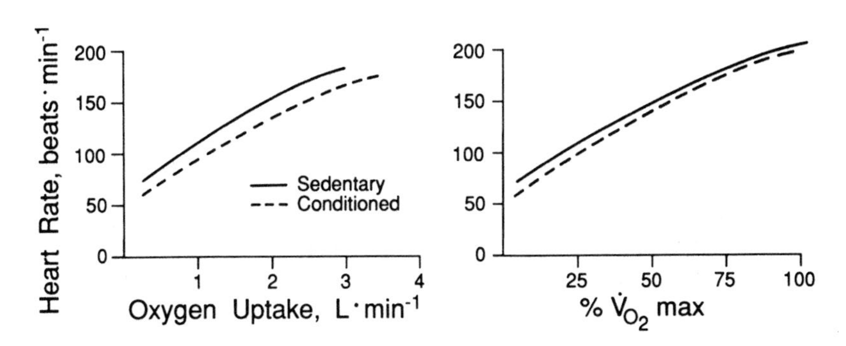

FIGURE 2–2. Relationship between heart rate and exercise intensity.

Considerable variability (±15 beats·min^{-1}) is associated with this estimate of maximal heart rate.

Following aerobic conditioning, resting heart rate is reduced by approximately 10 to 15 beats·min^{-1}. This is primarily attributed to enhanced parasympathetic tone. Decreased sympathetic discharge and a decrease in the intrinsic firing rate of the SA node may also contribute to the reduction in heart rate. Similarly, heart rate at any absolute submaximal oxygen uptake is significantly reduced. Maximal heart rate is unchanged or only slightly reduced after aerobic conditioning.

Stroke Volume

Stroke volume is the average volume of blood ejected per heart beat and is affected by various hemodynamic determinants. Left ventricular stroke volume is increased as a result of augmented diastolic filling (preload) via the Frank-Starling mechanism and is reduced by increased arterial blood pressure as well as other factors which raise impedance to aortic blood flow (afterload). Stroke volume is also increased by enhanced myocardial contractility, defined as the quality of ventricular performance at a constant level of ventricular preload, afterload and heart rate. Increased contractility results in an augmented ejection fraction or percent of end-diastolic volume ejected (stroke volume/end-diastolic volume) when heart rate and wall stress are held constant. Myocardial contractility is increased primarily by increased sympathetic neural stimulation of the left ventricle. Left ventricular contractile performance is also increased in conjunction with augmented heart rate (force-frequency relation). In the resting state, stroke volume is approximately 20% higher in the supine vs. upright posture as a result of greater venous return and is accompanied by a lower heart rate.

In the transition from rest to exercise in the upright posture, stroke volume rises primarily due to greater sympathetic neural stimulation and myocardial contractility, resulting in an increase in ejection fraction. An augmented end-diastolic volume as a consequence of increased venous return may also contribute to the rise in stroke volume at the onset of aerobic exercise.

Peak stroke volume during upright exercise is usually observed at approximately 40 to 50% of $\dot{V}O_{2max}$ (Fig. 2–3). A plateau in stroke volume at higher relative exercise intensities is usually observed due to the offsetting influences of increased

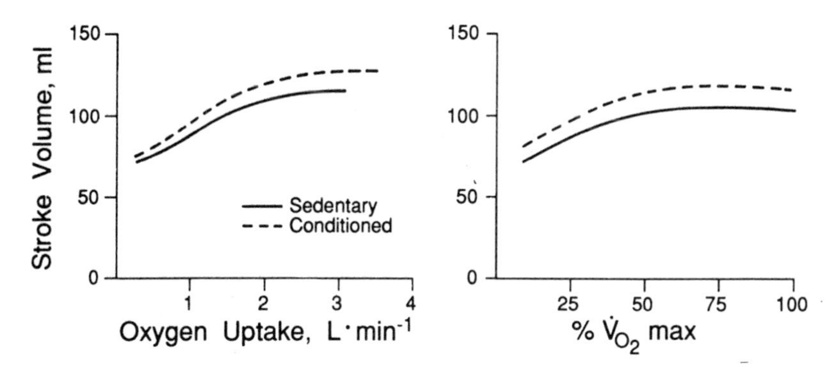

FIGURE 2–3. Relationship between stroke volume and exercise intensity.

myocardial contractility and ejection fraction and a progressive reduction in diastolic filling time as heart rate increases.

In healthy subjects, aerobic conditioning results in significant increases in stroke volume measured at rest, during submaximal exercise, and at maximal exercise. Although the mechanisms are not completely understood, current evidence indicates that the increase in maximal stroke volume is due primarily to reduced peripheral vascular resistance and enhanced preload. Changes in myocardial contractility and indices of systolic performance appear to be of lesser importance.

Cardiac Output

Cardiac output ($\dot{Q}$) rises linearly as a function of oxygen uptake or power output during submaximal exercise as a result of increases in heart rate and stroke volume (Fig. 2–4). Values for cardiac output peak immediately prior to the attainment of maximal oxygen uptake during graded exercise testing.

Aerobic conditioning of healthy individuals results in a significant increase in cardiac output measured at maximal exercise or at any given percent of $\dot{V}O_{2max}$ due to an increase in maximal stroke volume. As a result of the offsetting influences of reduced heart rate and augmented stroke volume, cardiac output measured at rest or any absolute submaximal oxygen uptake is not greatly altered by conditioning.

Blood Pressure

Blood pressure is the product of cardiac output and peripheral vascular resistance. Systolic pressure rises in a linear fash-

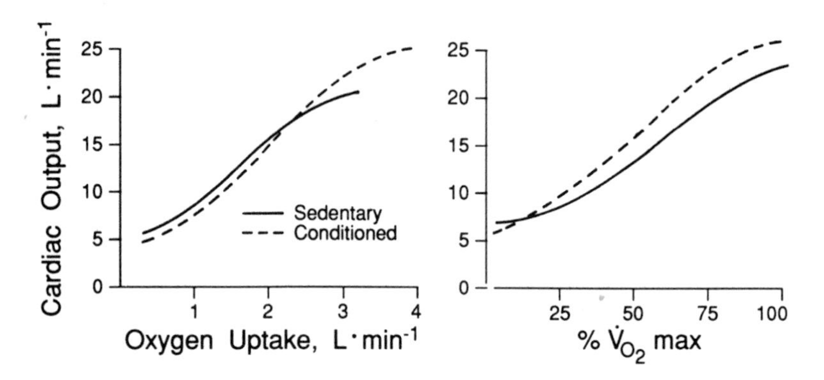

FIGURE 2–4. Relationship between cardiac output and exercise intensity.

ion as a function of exercise intensity, but diastolic pressure either falls moderately or remains unchanged from resting values. Therefore, pulse pressure (systolic blood pressure minus diastolic blood pressure) widens and mean blood pressure rises moderately with increasing exercise intensity in healthy individuals. Blood pressure at rest or at any given percent of $\dot{V}O_{2max}$ may be reduced moderately in healthy individuals following physical conditioning.

BLOOD FLOW REDISTRIBUTION

At rest 15 to 20% of the total cardiac output is distributed to the muscles and the remainder is channeled to other tissues, particularly the viscera. During exercise, blood flow is shunted away from the viscera and as much as 85% of the total cardiac output is directed toward exercising muscle.

During exercise, absolute coronary blood flow increases in proportion to cardiac output, but remains the same on a percentage basis (4 to 5% of total $\dot{Q}$). Absolute blood flow to the brain is slightly increased. Skin blood flow decreases at the onset of exercise due to augmented sympathetic activity. As exercise intensity increases, cutaneous blood flow rises as a result of sympathetic withdrawal in order to facilitate heat dissipation. During maximal or near maximal exercise, skin blood flow decreases to meet rising demands for blood flow from contracting skeletal muscle. During post-exercise recovery, skin blood flow again increases to facilitate heat dissipation.

Regulation of blood flow redistribution is achieved by the complex interaction of local metabolic and central autonomic nervous functions. The result of this interaction is a progressive decline in systemic vascular resistance during exercise of increasing intensity.

OXYGEN UTILIZATION

Oxygen uptake by skeletal muscle as reflected by the arteriovenous oxygen difference ($a-\bar{v}O_2$) increases progressively as a function of exercise intensity (Fig. 2–5).

Oxygen extraction depends on the oxygen content of arterial blood, the extent of redistribution of cardiac output, and the rate of oxygen removal by skeletal muscle and other tissues. The latter depends on muscle capillarity, myoglobin content, mitochondrial number and size and the oxidative capacity of mitochondrial enzymes. Therefore, the ratio of type I/type II motor units can alter the rate of oxygen utilization by skeletal muscle.

The content of arterial blood both at rest and during exercise is approximately 20 $ml \cdot 100ml^{-1}$. In the transition from rest to maximal exercise, $a-\bar{v}O_2$ increases from approximately 5 to 16 $ml \cdot 100ml^{-1}$. During maximal exercise, approximately 85% of the oxygen is removed from the blood perfusing skeletal muscle. A small percentage of the total cardiac output continues to perfuse nonexercising tissues which do not have a high regional $a-\bar{v}O_2$. Therefore, at maximal exercise mixed venous blood is not completely deoxygenated.

Aerobic conditioning results in changes which can significantly increase the ability of skeletal muscle to utilize oxygen.

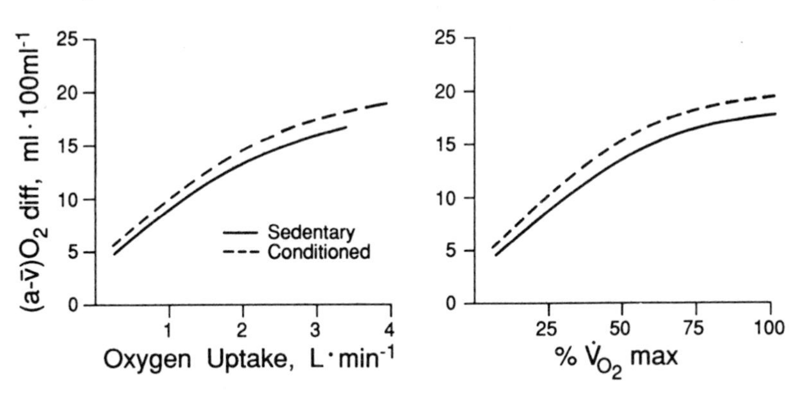

FIGURE 2–5. Relationship between arteriovenous oxygen difference and exercise intensity.

These include greater capillary density, increased mitochondrial size and density, enhanced oxidative enzyme activities and increased myoglobin content. Total muscle blood flow is increased, but the rate of perfusion per kilogram of active muscle is not altered.

EXPRESSION OF EXERCISE DATA

Interpretation of physiological responses to acute exercise and to physical conditioning depends on how the data are expressed. Data obtained during exercise tolerance tests are usually plotted against either power output or oxygen uptake. As described above, a close predictable relationship usually exists between *absolute* values for power output (watts or $kg\text{-}m \cdot min^{-1}$) and the *absolute* rate of oxygen uptake ($l \cdot min^{-1}$). When one is interested in studying physiological responses to standard exercise tasks, expression of data as a function of absolute power output or oxygen uptake is most appropriate.

Aerobic conditioning results in a significant reduction in the magnitude of variables such as heart rate, blood pressure, lactate production, and rating of perceived exertion (RPE; see Chapter 4) at any given submaximal power output. Such variables are regulated as a function of relative (percent of maximal) power output or oxygen uptake. Also, the magnitude of aerobic conditioning responses is related closely to the percent of functional capacity employed in conditioning sessions. Therefore, such variables are often employed for the prescription of exercise intensity (Fig. 2–6).

QUANTIFICATION OF EXERCISE RESPONSES (THE FICK EQUATION)

The physiologic processes that contribute to oxygen transport and utilization are described above. From a mathematical viewpoint, these processes and their interrelationships can be quantified in accordance with the Fick equation expressed in the following form:

$$\dot{V}O_2 = \dot{Q} \times a-\bar{v}O_2$$
$$\dot{Q} = HR \times SV$$

where:
$\dot{Q}$ = cardiac output
HR = heart rate
SV = stroke volume
$a-\bar{v}O_2$ = arteriovenous O_2 difference

Values observed during exercise tolerance testing vary depending on the individual's age, sex, body size, as well as the exercise modality and intensity. Approximate average data for young healthy adults of both sexes during weight-supported isotonic leg exercise (cycling) are provided in Table 2–4.

FUNCTIONAL LIMITATIONS IN DISEASE STATES

MYOCARDIAL ISCHEMIA

Myocardial ischemia is a state in which myocardial oxygen demand exceeds supply. From a functional viewpoint, ischemia

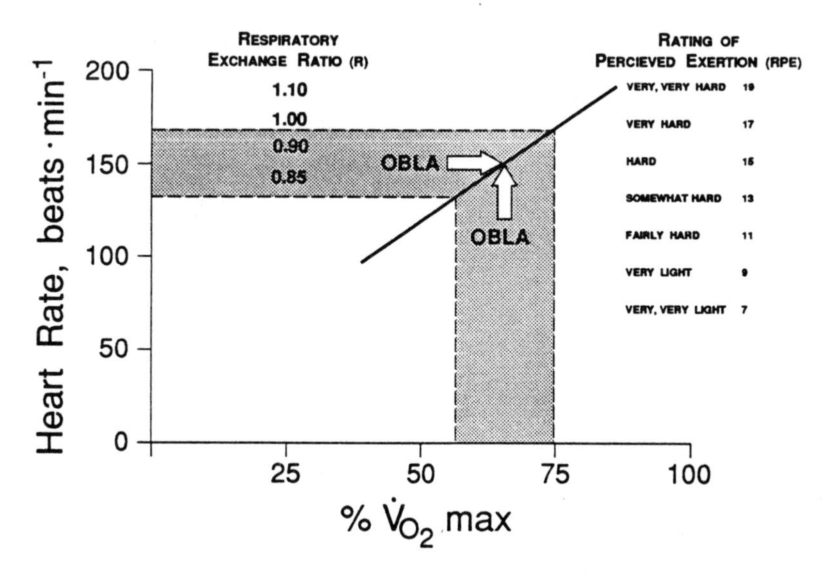

FIGURE 2–6. Interrelationships between indices of exercise intensity. Adapted from Hellerstein and Franklin.[13] Hellerstein HK and Franklin BA: Exercise testing and prescription. In *Rehabilitation of the Coronary Patient,* 2nd Ed. Edited by NK Wenger and HK Hellerstein. New York: John Wiley and Sons, 1984.

Table 2–4. Typical Responses to Graded Exercise in Healthy Adults.

Conditioning State	Intensity	% Maximum	$\dot{V}O_2$ (L·min^{-1})	HR (beats·min^{-1})	SV (ml·beat^{-1})	$\dot{Q}$ (L·min^{-1})	$a-\bar{v}O_2$ (ml·100ml^{-1})
A. *Young Men* (Weight, 75 kg)							
Untrained	Rest	—	0.30	70	85	5.95	5.0
Trained		—	0.30	55	100	5.5	5.5
Untrained	300 kg-	28	1.00	110	95	10.5	9.5
Trained	min^{-1} (50 watts)	23	1.00	100	105	10.5	9.5
Untrained	600 kg-	46	1.60	130	105	13.5	12.0
Trained	min^{-1} (100 watts)	38	1.60	115	115	13.4	12.0
Untrained	900 kg-	65	2.30	150	110	16.5	14.0
Trained	min^{-1} (150 watts)	53	2.30	130	125	16.3	14.2
Untrained	Maximal	100	3.25	195	110	21.5	15.0
Trained	Exercise	100	4.00	195	128	25.0	16.0
B. *Young Women* (Weight, 55 kg)							
Untrained	Rest	—	0.23	70	65	4.5	5.0
Trained		—	0.23	55	75	4.1	5.5
Untrained	200 kg-	33	0.75	110	75	8.3	9.0
Trained	min^{-1} (33 watts)	27	0.75	100	85	9.0	9.0
Untrained	400 kg-	51	1.15	135	80	10.8	10.5
Trained	min^{-1} (66 watts)	42	1.15	120	90	10.8	10.5
Untrained	600 kg-	69	1.55	155	85	13.2	12.0
Trained	min^{-1} (100 watts)	56	1.55	135	95	13.0	11.6
Untrained	Maximal	100	2.25	195	85	16.5	13.5
Trained	Exercise	100	2.75	195	98	19.0	14.5

leads to reduced myocardial contractility, altered electrical conduction, ventricular ectopic pacemaker activity, and in severe cases, chronic heart failure. Myocardial ischemia may be asymptomatic or may result in angina pectoris. Angina is discomfort, usually with a heavy, crushing quality, felt in the center of the chest, which often radiates down the left arm and to the neck and jaw. Shortness of breath and autonomic symptoms such as lightheadedness, nausea, or sweating may also be felt in conjunction with or as subjective equivalents of angina.

Determinants of myocardial oxygen uptake ($M\dot{V}O_2$) include heart rate, ventricular wall tension (preload and afterload), and contractility. Heart rate is the most important of these determinants and the rate-pressure product [(RPP), heart rate × systolic blood pressure × 10^{-2}] is often employed as an index of $M\dot{V}O_2$ during graded exercise testing.

Myocardial oxygen supply depends on the rate of coronary blood flow. Increased $M\dot{V}O_2$ during exercise is primarily the result of increased coronary blood flow with only a modest increase in the already substantial myocardial $a-\bar{v}O_2$ difference. Coronary blood flow occurs primarily during diastole and depends on the interaction between aortic diastolic blood pressure and coronary resistance. During exercise, the coronary vessels dilate as a result of local metabolic effects. $Beta_2$ adrenergic activity may also contribute to coronary vasodilation during exercise.

Factors which can reduce coronary blood flow in patients with coronary artery disease include coronary atherogenesis, coronary artery spasm, and acute coronary thrombosis. Coronary atherogenesis becomes physiologically important when approximately 60 to 75% of the vessel cross-sectional area is obstructed. The causes of coronary artery spasm are not completely understood, but spasm can result in myocardial ischemia both in the presence or absence of significant coronary atherogenic obstruction. Aggregation of platelets is thought to be involved as an important step in thrombus formation.

BED REST EFFECTS

Bed rest associated with disease, surgery, or medical treatment can result in significant decrements in physiological functions. These effects may add to limitations imposed by pathological conditions, resulting in marked reductions in physical performance capacities.

$\dot{V}O_{2max}$ decreases up to 25% with prolonged bed rest, primarily as a result of reduced plasma volume, red cell mass, stroke volume, and maximal exercise cardiac output. The oxidative capacity of skeletal muscle also decreases, resulting in reduced capacity for submaximal exercise. Maximal $a-\bar{v}O_2$ difference, however, is not greatly altered. Orthostatic tolerance can be reduced markedly due to reduced circulating blood volume and decrements in vasomotor function. Heat tolerance is also reduced.

Effects of prolonged bed rest on skeletal muscle include a negative nitrogen balance, atrophy, loss of tone and loss of muscular strength and endurance. Other undesirable effects include bone demineralization, reduced insulin sensitivity and carbohydrate tolerance, increased serum lipids, altered immune system function and greater susceptibility to renal infection, deep vein thrombosis, and sleep disturbances.

Unless dictated by severe disease, surgery or other compelling reasons, sustained bed rest is physiologically debilitating and should be avoided. In this regard, current medical practice involves early ambulation during recovery from acute illness or surgery.

OTHER PATHOPHYSIOLOGICAL CONSIDERATIONS

In addition to myocardial ischemia, functional capacity and its determinants can be altered by a wide range of pathophysiological and pharmacological factors. An in-depth discussion of each of these variables is beyond the scope of this chapter but examples are provided in Table 2–5.

FUNCTIONAL AEROBIC IMPAIRMENT

As summarized in Table 2–5, functional capacity can be reduced by many clinical conditions. In rehabilitative exercise settings it is important to be able to quantify the degree of disability resulting from such conditions and also to measure reductions in disability that may result from medical, surgical or rehabilitative interventions. In response to this need, Bruce

Table 2–5. Some Clinical and Physiological Factors That Can Reduce Determinants of Functional Capacity ($\dot{V}O_{2max}$).

Maximum Heart Rate	*Maximum Stroke Volume*	*Arterial O_2 Content*	*Mixed Venous O_2 Content*
Aging	Bed rest	Chronic obstructive pulmonary disease	Malnutrition
Coronary artery disease	Coronary heart disease	Interstitial lung disease	Muscular dystrophy
AV heart block	Cardiomyopathy	Anemia	
Sick sinus syndrome	Valvular heart disease	Hemoglobinopathy	
Advanced pregnancy	Severe hypertension	Smoking	
Cardiomyopathy	Congestive heart failure		
Beta-adrenergic blockade	Advanced pregnancy		
Congestive heart failure			
Autonomic dysfunction			

and colleagues[3] developed the concept of Functional Aerobic Impairment (FAI):

$$\text{Percentage FAI} = \frac{\text{Predicted } \dot{V}O_{2max} - \text{Observed } \dot{V}O_{2max}}{\text{Predicted } \dot{V}O_{2max}} \times 10^{-2}$$

Where: Observed $\dot{V}O_{2max}$ = the individual's $\dot{V}O_{2max}$ ($ml \cdot kg^{-1} \cdot min^{-1}$) measured during exercise tolerance testing

Predicted $\dot{V}O_{2max}$ = an average value for healthy individuals of the same age, sex, and activity level

FAI is essentially the percentage that an individual's functional capacity falls below that expected for his/her age, sex, and conditioning state. For example, an FAI score of 0 indicates achievement of predicted functional capacity. Predicted $\dot{V}O_{2max}$ ($ml \cdot kg^{-1} \cdot min^{-1}$) can be predicted using the following regression equations:

Active men:	69.7—0.612 age (yr)
Active women:	42.9—0.312 age (yr)
Sedentary men:	57.8—0.445 age (yr)
Sedentary women:	42.3—0.356 age (yr)

Values for FAI can be described according to the following qualitative scale:

0–26%	No significant FAI
27–40%	Mild impairment
41–54%	Moderate impairment
55–68%	Marked impairment
>68%	Extreme impairment

*Note that negative values for FAI indicate that functional capacity is above average.

SPECIAL EXERCISE CONDITIONS

DYNAMIC (ISOTONIC) ARM EXERCISE

Relative to leg ergometry, isotonic exercise performed using the arms and shoulders involves a smaller muscle mass and the $\dot{V}O_{2max}$ of arm cranking exercise is approximately 60 to 70% of $\dot{V}O_{2max}$ measured during analogous leg exercise. During submaximal exercise, both oxygen uptake and cardiac output are proportional to the mass of exercising muscle in both arm and leg exercise. Therefore, the ratio of cardiac output to oxygen uptake is similar (approximately 6 L blood flow/L oxygen uptake). Blood flow to the skin and nonexercising tissues relates more closely to either percent $\dot{V}O_{2max}$ or heart rate than absolute oxygen uptake.

During arm vs. leg exercise at any given power output or percent $\dot{V}O_{2max}$, heart rate is higher and stroke volume is lower during arm cranking. The smaller stroke volume during arm exercise is due to a lower rate of venous return from venous capacitance vessels in the noncontracting lower extremities. Also, systolic and diastolic blood pressures are higher during arm vs. leg exercise at any given absolute power output or percent $\dot{V}O_{2max}$ as a result of factors that lead to a higher systemic vascular resistance during arm exercise.[4]

Maximal heart rate may be somewhat lower during maximal arm vs. leg ergometry because the metabolic capacity of a smaller contracting muscle mass limits exercise performance relative to that seen with corresponding leg exercise.

INTERMITTENT EXERCISE

Intermittent exercise involves alternating periods of work and rest. The main advantage of this type of exercise is that it can allow the performance of a greater total volume of high intensity exercise (intensity > OBLA) than continuous exercise of the same intensity. In this regard, the anaerobic ATP-CP system is utilized at the beginning of high intensity exertion prior to engagement of anaerobic glycolysis. Thus, if the work interval is sufficiently short and if the subsequent rest period is long enough to permit replenishment of ATP-CP stores, then significant muscle and blood lactate accumulation can be prevented.

To avoid fatigue, the work:rest ratio must usually be kept less than 1:3 if the exercise is heavy. However, the lower the intensity of work, the longer the exercise period and shorter the rest interval can be. This will also change the energy systems that are being conditioned. In general, a work:rest ratio of approximately 1:3, with a brief (< 10 seconds) intensive exercise interval will effectively train the ATP-CP anaerobic system. Anaerobic glycolysis is stressed to a greater extent when the work period is 45 to 90 seconds long and the work:rest ratio is approximately 1:2. Finally, a longer (≥ 2 minutes), less intense work period and work:rest ratio of approximately 1:1 is more useful to train the aerobic metabolic pathways. In the latter type of exercise, the recovery interval is shorter relative to the exercise interval so that complete recovery of the oxygen transport system does not occur.

ISOMETRIC (STATIC) EXERCISE

Physiologic responses to isometric exercise differ from those of dynamic (isotonic) exercise in several fundamental ways. First, it is most convenient to quantify the intensity of such exercise as a percentage of maximum voluntary contraction (MVC). In this regard, isometric exertion is primarily anaerobic in nature since oxygen delivery is minimized due to sustained compression of the arterial vessels by muscle contraction. Isometric exercise above approximately 15% MVC results in complete occlusion of arterial blood flow and leads to muscular fatigue. The time to muscular fatigue is inversely proportional to the percent MVC.

The cardiovascular effects of isometric exercise are referred to as the "pressor response." This is a reflex response to metabolic events in ischemic muscle. The magnitude of physiological changes depends on both the percent MVC and the muscle mass involved in the exercise. The pressor response involves only moderate increases in oxygen uptake, heart rate, and cardiac output relative to isotonic exercise. Also, there is little or no change in either stroke volume or systemic vascular resistance. However, arterial blood pressure (particularly diastolic) and the rate-pressure product (RPP) increase markedly (Table 2–6). Despite this significant rise in the RPP, isometric exercise

Table 2–6. Comparison of Cardiovascular Responses to High Intensity Static vs. Dynamic Exercise.

	Magnitude of Change from Rest to Exercise	
Variable	*Static*	*Dynamic*
Oxygen uptake	↑	↑ ↑ ↑
Heart rate	↑	↑ ↑ ↑
Stroke volume	±	↑ ↑
Cardiac output	↑	↑ ↑ ↑
Peripheral vascular resistance	±	↓
Systolic blood pressure	↑	↑ ↑
Diastolic blood pressure	↑ ↑ ↑	±
Rate-pressure product	↑ ↑ ↑	↑ ↑ ↑
Left ventricular Wall stress	Primarily pressure loading	Primarily volume loading

is less likely than isotonic exercise to provoke angina pectoris in patients with coronary artery disease perhaps as a result of enhanced coronary blood flow during diastole.

Blood pressure responses to isometric exercise are significantly altered by the Valsalva maneuver, which involves forced expiration against a closed glottis during exertional straining. Initially, arterial blood pressure is increased since the maneuver augments intrathoracic pressure and this in turn raises aortic blood pressure. During sustained exertion, arterial blood pressure declines as a consequence of reduced venous return and cardiac output due to compression of the large veins. Subsequently, the fall in blood pressure leads to reduced arterial baroreceptor activity and reflex-mediated increases in both heart rate and systemic vascular resistance. On cessation of exertion, venous return and cardiac output are quickly restored, but systemic vascular resistance remains high causing temporary elevation of blood pressure. Heart rate is again reduced by baroreceptor-mediated cardiovascular reflex activity.

SUMMARY

Three major systems provide energy for the performance of physical exercise: stored phosphagens (ATP, CP), anaerobic glycolysis, and oxidative metabolism. The most important energy system for sustained exercise is the oxidative system. Maximal aerobic power ($\dot{V}O_{2max}$) depends on several essential processes: pulmonary ventilation, alveolar-arterial gas exchange, cardiac output, blood flow redistribution, and oxygen utilization by skeletal muscle. These metabolic and cardiopulmonary processes can be expressed mathematically according to the Fick equation.

Maximal oxygen uptake and its determinants can be altered by several variables including sex, body size, environmental conditions, and various cardiopulmonary diseases. In particular, disease conditions which result in reduced myocardial oxygen supply or increased demand can lead to myocardial ischemia and impaired cardiac performance. $\dot{V}O_{2max}$ is also reduced significantly by chronic bed rest and increased by aerobic-type conditioning.

Metabolic and cardiorespiratory responses to exercise vary with the type of exercise being performed. Dynamic arm (vs. leg) exercise is characterized by a higher heart rate and lower stroke volume at any given submaximal power output. $\dot{V}O_{2max}$

during arm exercise is approximately 70% of that for dynamic leg exercise. Use of an intermittent exercise protocol allows the completion of more high intensity exercise compared to continuous exercise of the same intensity since blood lactate accumulation is avoided or delayed. Finally, strenuous static (vs. dynamic) exercise results in a moderate increase in heart rate, no reduction in peripheral vascular resistance and substantial increases in blood pressure (particularly diastolic).

REFERENCES

1. Åstrand P-O and Rodahl K: *Textbook of Work Physiology,* 3rd ed. New York: McGraw-Hill, 1986.
2. Brooks FA and Fahey TD: *Exercise Physiology: Human Bioenergetics and its Applications.* New York: John Wiley and Sons, 1984.
3. Bruce RA, Kusumi F and Hosmer D: Maximal oxygen intake and homographic assessment of functional aerobic impairment in cardiovascular disease. *Am Heart J 85*:546–562, 1973.
4. Clausen JP: Circulatory adjustments to dynamic exercise and effect of physical training in normal subjects and in patients with coronary artery disease. *Prog Cardiovasc Dis 28*:459–495, 1976.
5. Dehn MM, Blomqvist GG and Mitchell JH: Clinical exercise performance. *Clin Sports Med 3*:319–332, 1984.
6. Durstine JL and Pate RR: Cardiorespiratory responses to acute exercise. In American College of Sports Medicine, *Resource Manual for Guidelines for Exercise Testing and Prescription.* Philadelphia: Lea & Febiger, 1988.
7. Fox EL and Mathews DK: *The Physiological Bases of Physical Education and Athletics.* Philadelphia: W.B. Saunders Co., 1981.
8. Franklin BA, Gordon S and Timmins GC: Fundamentals of exercise physiology: Implications for exercise testing and prescription. In *Exercise in Modern Medicine.* Edited by BA Franklin, S Gordon and GC Timmins. Baltimore: Williams & Wilkins, 1989.
9. Frontera WR and Adams RP: Endurance exercise: Normal physiology and limitations imposed by pathological processes (Part 1). *Phys Sportsmed 14*:94–106, 1986.
10. Frontera WR and Adams RP: Endurance exercise: Normal physiology and limitations imposed by pathological processes (Part 2). *Phys Sportsmed 14*:103–120, 1986.
11. Hanson P: Pathophysiology of chronic diseases and exercise training. In *Resource Manual For Guidelines For Exercise Testing and Prescription.* Edited by American College of Sports Medicine. Philadelphia: Lea & Febiger, 1988.
12. Hanson P: Clinical exercise testing. In *Resource Manual For Guidelines For Exercise Testing and Prescription.* Edited by American College of Sports Medicine. Philadelphia: Lea & Febiger, 1988.
13. Hellerstein HK and Franklin BA: Exercise testing and prescription. In *Rehabilitation of the Coronary Patient,* 2nd Ed. Edited by NK Wenger and HK Hellerstein. New York: John Wiley and Sons, 1984.
14. Jones NL: *Clinical Exercise Testing,* 3rd Ed. Philadelphia: W.B. Saunders Co., 1988.

15. Knuttgen H: Force, work, power and exercise. *Med Sci Sports Exerc 10*:227–228, 1978.
16. McKirnan MD and Froelicher VF: General principles of exercise testing. In *Exercise Testing and Exercise Prescription for Special Cases.* Edited by JS Skinner. Philadelphia: Lea & Febiger, 1987.
17. Park CR and Crawford MH. Heart of the athlete. *Current Problems Cardiol 10*:1–73, 1985.
18. Wasserman K and Whipp BJ: Exercise physiology in health and disease. *Am Rev Resp Dis 112*:219–249, 1975.

CHAPTER 3

Physical Fitness Testing

The term "physical fitness" has been defined in many ways. Most definitions of physical fitness refer strictly to the capacity for movement and the following recently proposed definition is typical in this regard: *A set of attributes that people have or achieve that relates to the ability to perform physical activity.*[13] Such definitions are, by nature, rather broad and can be interpreted as encompassing an array of fitness components, some of which relate to athletic performance, but not health. Accordingly, the term "health-related physical fitness" has been used to denote fitness as it pertains to disease prevention and health promotion. One definition of health-related physical fitness is: *A state characterized by (a) an ability to perform daily activities with vigor, and (b) demonstration of traits and capacities that are associated with low risk of premature development of the hypokinetic diseases (i.e., those associated with physical inactivity).*[38]

Although many different literal definitions of physical fitness have developed, there is relative uniformity in the *operational* definition of physical fitness. It has almost always been viewed as a multifactorial construct that includes several components. Each component is a movement-related trait or capacity that is considered to be largely independent of the others. Health-related physical fitness is typically operationally defined as including cardiorespiratory endurance, body composition, muscular strength and endurance, and flexibility. The concept that underlies *health-related physical fitness* is that better status in each of the constituent components is associated with lower risk for development of disease and/or functional disability.

Measurement of physical fitness is a common and appropriate practice in preventive and rehabilitative exercise programs. The purposes of fitness testing in such programs include:

1. Provision of data that are helpful in development of exercise prescriptions,
2. Collection of baseline and follow-up data that allow evaluation of progress in program participants,
3. Motivation of participants by establishing reasonable and attainable fitness goals,
4. Education of participants concerning the concept of physical fitness and individual fitness status.

A fundamental goal of preventive and rehabilitative exercise programs is promotion of health. Therefore, such programs should, and usually do, focus on enhancement of the health-related components of physical fitness. This chapter provides guidelines for the measurement and evaluation of health-related physical fitness and for health screening of participants before administration of a physical fitness test.

PRE-PARTICIPATION HEALTH SCREENING

Programs to enhance health-related fitness are usually conducted in nonmedical settings and the majority of prospective participants are apparently healthy adults whose goals are to maintain health and enhance health-related fitness components. Accordingly, in such settings the purposes of pre-participation health screening are the following:

1. To identify and exclude individuals with medical contraindications to exercise,
2. To identify persons with clinically significant disease conditions who should be referred to a medically supervised exercise program,
3. To identify individuals with disease symptoms and risk factors for disease development who should receive further medical evaluation before starting an exercise program, and
4. To identify persons with special needs for safe exercise participation (e.g., elderly persons, pregnant women).

In most fitness programs, it is essential that health screening procedures be both valid and cost-effective. Also, procedures should also be time-efficient so that unnecessary barriers to participation are avoided. Available health screening devices listed in increasing order of cost and complexity include the following:

1. Self-administered health questionnaires
2. Physical examination by a physician
3. Analysis of CAD risk profile
4. Diagnostic exercise testing
5. Advanced cardiac diagnostic tests (e.g., ^{201}thallium imaging, coronary angiography)

As outlined in Chapter 1, it is recommended that apparently healthy men greater than 40 years of age and apparently healthy women greater than age 50 have a medical examination and diagnostic exercise test before starting a *vigorous* exercise program. However, these procedures are not essential when such persons begin a *moderate* intensity exercise regimen.

Pre-participation screening of asymptomatic men under age 40 and women under age 50 for vigorous exercise and of apparently healthy individuals of any age for moderate exercise can be effectively and efficiently accomplished using validated self-administered questionnaires. A widely utilized example of such an instrument is the Physical Activity Readiness Questionnaire (PAR-Q, see Table 3–1). The PAR-Q was developed in Canada by the British Columbia Ministry of Health. It was first made available in 1978 and has been used as a pretest screening instrument prior to administration of the Canadian

Table 3–1. Physical Activity Readiness Questionnaire.*

For most people, physical activity should not pose any problem or hazard. PAR-Q has been designed to identify the small number of adults for whom physical activity might be inappropriate or those who should have medical advice concerning the type of activity most suitable.

1. Has your doctor ever said you have heart trouble?
2. Do you frequently suffer from pains in your chest?
3. Do you often feel faint or have spells of severe dizziness?
4. Has a doctor ever said your blood pressure was too high?
5. Has a doctor ever told you that you have a bone or joint problem such as arthritis that has been aggravated by exercise, or might be made worse with exercise?
6. Is there a good physical reason not mentioned here why you should not follow an activity program even if you wanted to?
7. Are you over age 65 and not accustomed to vigorous exercise?

If a person answers yes to any question, vigorous exercise or exercise testing should be postponed. Medical clearance may be necessary.

*Reference: PAR-Q Validation Report. British Columbia Department of Health, June 1975 (Modified Version).

Aerobic Fitness Test (formerly Canadian Home Fitness Test) for over 1 million people, none of whom have experienced any serious cardiovascular problems. It is essentially 100% sensitive for the detection of medical contraindications to exercise and approximately 80% specific. Its ability to predict subsequent exercise ECG abnormalities is less impressive, with a sensitivity and specificity of approximately 35 and 80%, respectively.[45] In Ontario, Canada, the PAR-Q has been recommended as a minimum pre-activity screening standard for entry into low to moderate intensity physical activity programs.[19]

A second screening instrument, the Physical Activity Readiness Examination (PAR-X) was later developed in order to facilitate medical examinations resulting from positive responses to the PAR-Q. It includes a checklist of recommended procedures for use in pre-activity medical examinations, and incorporates a Physical Activity Prescription form (PAR_x). The latter form lists absolute and relative contraindication to exercise, includes a summary of guidelines for exercise prescription and provides special prescriptive advice for use in conjunction with common medical, pharmacological, and environmental conditions. An important feature of this form is that it aids in the education of physicians who may not be familiar with the principles of pre-activity screening and exercise prescription. Copies of the PAR-Q and PAR-X can be obtained by writing:

Government of Canada
Fitness and Amateur Sport
365 Laurier Avenue West
Ottawa, Ontario CANADA K1A 0X6

Despite the advantages cited above for the PAR-Q, several limitations to its use have been identified.[19] First, its limited specificity for detecting contraindications to exercise results primarily from false positive answers to the question, "Has a doctor ever said that your blood pressure was too high?". Second, the question "Are you over age 65 and not accustomed to vigorous exercise?" may fail to screen out some individuals with premature aging effects. Conversely, apparently healthy persons over age 65 who wish to participate in mild to moderate exercise may be discouraged or inappropriately inconvenienced by an automatic referral for medical clearance by a physician. Finally, there is no provision on the PAR-Q form to identify pregnant women or individuals on prescription medication which may alter the safety of exercise. Thus, the PAR-Q should be used by fitness professionals with these limitations in mind.

CARDIORESPIRATORY ENDURANCE

Cardiorespiratory endurance (CRE) is defined as the ability to perform large-muscle, dynamic, moderate-to-high intensity exercise for prolonged periods. Performance of such exercise depends on the functional state of the respiratory, cardiovascular, and skeletal muscle systems. Cardiorespiratory endurance is considered health-related because: (a) low levels of fitness have been associated with markedly increased risk of premature death from all causes and from cardiovascular disease specifically, and (b) higher fitness is associated with higher levels of habitual physical activity which is, in turn, associated with many health benefits.

The traditionally accepted criterion measure of cardiorespiratory endurance is directly measured maximal oxygen consumption ($\dot{V}O_{2max}$). Direct measurement of $\dot{V}O_{2max}$ involves analysis of expired air samples collected while the subject performs graded, maximal exercise. Detailed descriptions of recommended procedures for direct measurement of $\dot{V}O_{2max}$ are provided elsewhere.[25] For the purpose of evaluating CRE, $\dot{V}O_{2max}$ values are typically expressed relative to body weight (i.e., $ml \cdot kg^{-1} \cdot min^{-1}$).

Because direct measurement of $\dot{V}O_{2max}$ is often not feasible, many procedures for estimation of $\dot{V}O_{2max}$ have been developed. These tests have been validated by examining: (a) the correlation between directly measured $\dot{V}O_{2max}$ and estimated $\dot{V}O_{2max}$ determined from physiologic responses to submaximal exercise (e.g., heart rate at a specified power output), or (b) the correlation between directly measured $\dot{V}O_{2max}$ and test performance (e.g., mile run for time).

Following are concise descriptions of some of the more common approaches to assessment of cardiorespiratory endurance.

SUBMAXIMAL CYCLE ERGOMETER TESTS

An estimate of $\dot{V}O_{2max}$ can be derived from the heart rate response to standard submaximal exercise performed on a calibrated cycle ergometer. The procedure is based on the well-established linear relationship between heart rate and $\dot{V}O_2$ and on the fact that the maximal heart rate and $\dot{V}O_{2max}$ tend to be attained at similar rates of power output. Since cycle ergometer exercise is not a weight-bearing activity, absolute $\dot{V}O_2$ ($1 \cdot min^{-1}$) at a particular rate of power output is fairly similar in most persons (see Appendix D). However, body weight is a major determinant of the relative $\dot{V}O_2$ ($ml \cdot kg^{-1} \cdot min^{-1}$) during cycle exercise and individuals with greater muscle mass have a performance advantage. Therefore, in selecting rates of power output, modifications must be made for the individual's body weight.

There are several widely used submaximal cycle ergometer tests of cardiorespiratory endurance, and three of them will be described briefly. One of three protocols (Table 3–2) is selected according to the subject's weight and activity status as outlined in Table 3–3. Activity status is subjectively determined by the test administrator from reviewing questionnaire data provided by the participant or by verbal query. Individuals who have been regularly participating (the last 3 months) in vigorous activities for at least 15 minutes, 3 times per week, are classified as very active.

Exercise heart rates are monitored during the test by palpation of the pulse or by electronic monitoring. Heart rate is checked during the last 15 seconds of each test stage, and the test is terminated when the heart rate reaches 65 to 70% of the predicted age-adjusted maximal heart rate (Table 3–4). These percentages of maximal heart rate will be inaccurate in individuals

Table 3–2. Test Protocols.

	Test Stages (minutes)			
Protocol	*I (1–2)*	*II (3–4)*	*III (5–6)*	*IV (7–8)*
A	*25 (150)	50 (300)	75 (450)	100 (600)
B	25 (150)	50 (300)	100 (600)	150 (900)
C	50 (300)	100 (600)	150 (900)	200 (1200)

*Workload in watts (kilogram meters per minute)

Table 3–3. Protocol Selection Criteria.

Body Weight in kg (lbs)	*Very Active*	
	No	*Yes*
<73 (160)	A	A
74–90 (161–199)	A	B
>91 (200)	B	C

Table 3–4. Target Heart Rate for Cycle Ergometer.

Age (years)	*Heart Rate (beats/minute)*
<20	140
20–29	135
30–39	130
40–49	120
50–59	115
60–65	110

who are taking drugs which blunt the heart rate response to exercise (e.g., beta blockers).

Heart rate is measured for at least two and preferably three test stages. A rough estimate of $\dot{V}O_{2max}$ can then be extrapolated using the predicted age-adjusted maximal heart rate as illustrated in Figure 3–1.

The **YMCA Cycle Ergometer Test**[24] is similar to that just described except that workloads are selected using a "branching" protocol. The test begins with a power output of 150 $kp \cdot m \cdot min^{-1}$. After 3 minutes heart rate is measured and power output is increased by an amount that is inversely related to heart rate. Using the heart rates and power output for three stages, $\dot{V}O_{2max}$ is estimated by extrapolation.

The **Astrand-Rhyming Test**[5] is another cycle ergometer test used to estimate $\dot{V}O_{2max}$. It differs from those described above in that the estimated $\dot{V}O_{2max}$ is derived from the heart rate response to a single rate of power output. Test duration is 6 minutes and pedal revolutions are to be kept constant at 50 revolutions per minute. The designated power output is based on gender and activity history as follows:

	Power Output ($kp \cdot m \cdot min^{-1}$)
Unconditioned	
Males	300 or 600
Females	300 or 450
Conditioned	
Males	600 or 900
Females	450 or 650

Using the average heart rate measured during the last 10 seconds of the final 2 minutes and the power output, maximal oxygen uptake can be estimated.[4,26] This value must then be corrected using published correction factors.

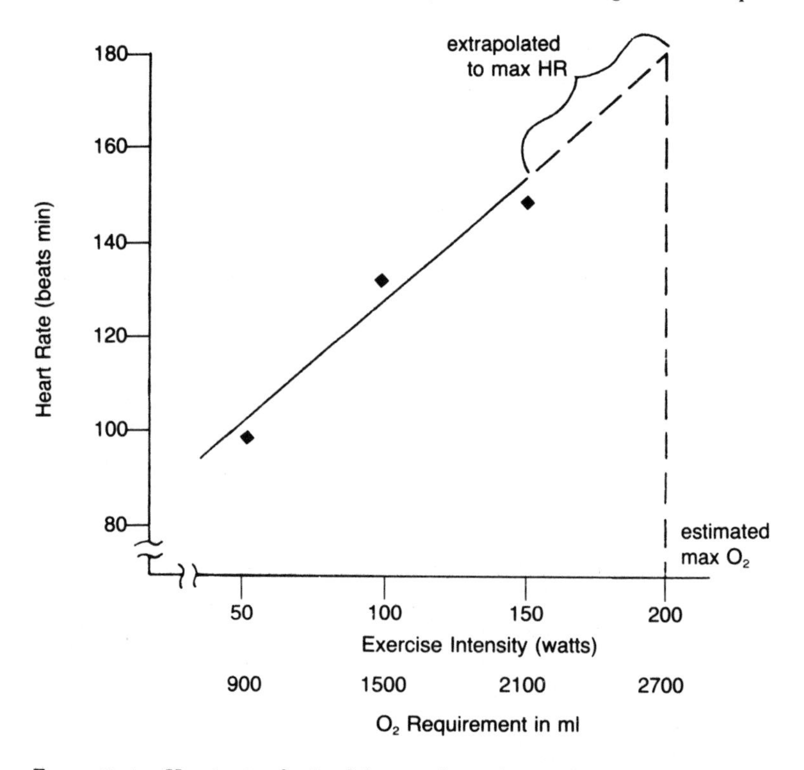

FIGURE 3–1. Heart rate obtained from at least three submaximal exercise intensities may be extrapolated to the age predicted maximal heart rate. A vertical line to the intensity scale estimates maximal exercise intensity. (Adapted from: Blair SN: *Behavioral Health: A Handbook of Health Enhancement and Disease Prevention.* Edited by JD Matarazzo, et al. New York: John Wiley & Sons, 1984, p. 438.)

STEP TESTS

The **3-Minute Step Test** is a test that has been used for mass testing. According to the YMCA protocol,[24] the test is to be conducted on a 12-inch high bench, with a stepping rate of 24 steps/minute for 3 minutes. After the test is completed, the subject is to immediately sit down and heart beats are counted for 1 minute. Counting must start within 5 seconds of the end of the test. Using this heart rate, a qualitative rating of fitness can be determined using a nomogram.[24]

DISTANCE RUNS

Various field tests of CRE can be employed when equipment is not available or mass testing is required. The **1.5 Mile Run**[6] is best suited for active individuals since it requires maximal effort. Participants are to run 1.5 miles on a level course as fast as possible after a light warm-up. Proper pacing and high motivation are required for best performance. $\dot{V}O_{2max}$ is estimated from the performance time recorded.[16,26]

The **12-Minute Run** is a similar test used to estimate $\dot{V}O_{2max}$. Participants are to run as far as possible in 12 minutes. The distance run is used to determine $\dot{V}O_{2max}$. Norms are available for males and females of various age groups.[26]

WALKING TESTS

The **1-Mile Walk Test** has been developed for adults, especially older adults. The test consists of a warm-up and a 1 mile walk as fast as possible. Only walking is allowed. Post-exercise heart rate and performance time are used to predict $\dot{V}O_{2max}$. Norm tables are available.[26]

The **Rockport Fitness Walking Test** has also been validated as a fitness test.[32] Participants walk 1 mile as fast as possible, record their time, and count their heart rate immediately after finishing. Generalized and gender-specific regression equations have been developed to estimate $\dot{V}O_{2max}$.[32]

BODY COMPOSITION

RATIONALE

Evaluation of body composition typically is included as part of a health screen or physical fitness assessment. It is well established that excess body fat is harmful to health, but there are many misconceptions about the assessment and interpretation of body composition. There has been a change in the cultural norm of ideal body composition over the past 2 or 3 decades. The slender bodies of movie stars and supermodels have become the ideal that many strive, usually unsuccessfully, to emulate. The U.S. National Center for Health Statistics surveys[37] show that nearly 50% of adult women in the U.S. report that they are dieting to lose weight. Only about 25% of women are at increased health risk because of overweight, according to standards established by the U.S. Surgeon General. Thus, twice as many women are dieting as can be justified by health reasons. The dieting mania is even more prevalent in teen-aged girls in the U.S. with 60 to 75% reporting that they are dieting to lose weight.

Some exercise professionals may have contributed to the extreme concern with thinness referred to above by subtly, or perhaps even directly, implying that with a little effort all exercise program participants can become slim. For several reasons such an implication is problematic. First, it ignores research studies. Exercise can help individuals lose weight, but it is unrealistic to expect all exercise class members to develop a thin figure. Second, exercise professionals have frequently established targets for body composition that are unrealistically low, in terms of health benefit. Thinner is not necessarily healthier, evidenced by similar mortality risk across a wide range of body composition values. Health risk increases significantly only at the upper end of the body composition distribution. Third, we frequently ignore the principle of variability. Humans vary widely on any trait you can measure, and body composition is no exception. The exercise professional must recognize this and take it into account in interpreting body composition data.

ASSESSMENT

Body composition refers to the percentage of body weight that is fat (% body fat) and its measurement is based on the assumption that body weight can be dichotomized into lean body weight and fat weight. Body composition can be measured in many ways, including both laboratory and field techniques. Different assessment techniques are briefly reviewed in this section. Specific instructions for obtaining measurements and calculating estimates of body fat are beyond the scope of this text, but references for these techniques will be provided.

The criterion measure for assessing body composition is **hydrostatic (underwater) weighing.**[10,49] The procedure is described elsewhere.[35] This technique is based on Archimedes' principle, which states that when a body is immersed in water, it will be buoyed up by a counterforce equal to the weight of the water displaced. Bone and muscle tissue are more dense than water, whereas fat tissue is less dense than water. Therefore, a person with more lean body mass for the same total body weight weighs more in water and has a higher body density and, thus, lower percentage of body fat. Residual volume of the lungs is also needed to calculate body density and can be measured directly or estimated. Body density can be derived from the following formula:

$$\text{Body Density} = \frac{\text{Weight in air}}{\text{Weight in air} - \text{weight in water/Density of water}}$$

$$- \text{Residual Volume}$$

Prediction equations are then used to convert body density into percent body fat. Two commonly used formulas are:

$$\text{BF\%} = (457/\text{Body Density}) - 414.2$$ [9]

$$\text{BF\%} = (495/\text{Body Density}) - 450$$ [47]

Although hydrostatic weighing is the gold standard, the technique requires special equipment, is expensive, complicated, time-consuming, and subject to great error if conducted improperly.

Anthropometric methods provide a more practical and less expensive alternative to estimate body composition and are commonly used in a clinical or nonlaboratory setting, however, are not as accurate as hydrostatic weighing. Anthropometry includes measures such as height, weight, circumferences, diameters, and skinfolds.

Skinfold thicknesses correlate fairly well with hydrostatic weighing. The principle behind this technique is that approximately one-half of stored body fat is located as subcutaneous fat, which is closely related to overall fat.[30,31] Various regression equations have been developed to predict body density from skinfold measurements.[27,40,50,51] However, it must be kept in mind that the regression equation used is specific to the population from which it was derived.[49] Following are two commonly used prediction equations for adult males and females:

MALES: (27)

$$\text{Body Density} = 1.1093800 - 0.0008267\,(X2) + 0.0000016\,(X2)^2 - 0.0002574\,(X3)$$

X2 = sum of chest, abdomen, and thigh skinfolds (mm)

X3 = age (years)

FEMALES: (28)

$$\text{Body Density} = 1.0994921 - 0.0009929\,(X4) + 0.0000023\,(X4)^2 - 0.0001392\,(X3)$$

X3 = age (years)

X4 = sum of triceps, suprailium, and thigh skinfolds (mm)

Proper procedures for skinfold measurements are described elsewhere.[35]

Several prediction equations have also been developed utilizing **circumference measurements** in combination with skinfold measures. Various limb and body girths are measured and used in equations that predict body density or lean body mass.[21,48]

The **Body Mass Index (BMI)**, or Quetelet index, is used to assess weight relative to height and is calculated by dividing body weight in kilograms by height in meters squared (wt/ht^2). BMI is a good indicator of total body composition in population-based studies and is related to health outcomes.

Excessive body fat is a health hazard. The distribution of body fat also is important. Persons with more fat on the trunk, especially abdominal fat, are at increased risk of death when compared to persons who are equally fat, but have more of their fat on the extremities. A simple measure that is associated with increased risk is the waist/hip ratio (circumference of the waist divided by the circumference of the hips).[8] Ratios above .95 for men and .85 for women are considered to place the person at significantly increased risk.

Many other methods are currently being used to assess body composition, however, more research is needed to establish their reliability and validity. These methods include ultrasound, which directly measures the depth of the adipose tissue and muscle; the measurement of total body water through the use of isotopically labeled water; infrared interactance which is based on the principles of light absorption, reflection, and near-infrared spectroscopy; and bioelectrical impedance which is based on the premise that water conducts electricity but fat does not, and therefore, total body water can be detected as a current is passed through the subject.[15,18,22]

INTERPRETATION OF BODY COMPOSITION MEASURES

Prospective epidemiological studies show a reverse "J" relationship between body fat and risk of death during a follow-up period.[37] The excess risk in the lean is thought to be due to pre-existing disease. Note that the relation between body composition and mortality is relatively flat across a wide range. Significant increases in risk begin at a BMI of about 27.8 kg/m^2 for men and 27.3 kg/m^2 for women. The message is that we should tolerate a broad range of body composition values as normal. Intensive intervention for weight loss should be implemented in persons at the upper end of the distribution.

Interpretation of a person's body composition must be individualized. The exercise professional should be aware of the wide range of normal values, and not encourage all participants to achieve a particular value. The individual's clinical status and other risk factors must be taken into account. For example, consider a 50-year-old man with an estimated body fat of 16%. This value is well within the range of normal espoused by most authorities. However, suppose that this man also has a total cholesterol of 285 $mg \cdot dl^{-1}$ and a blood pressure of 160/97. Appropriate advice to this man would be that, "Although your body composition is within the usual range of normal, you will probably benefit if you could lose 5 or 10 pounds. Your cholesterol and blood pressure are high, and we know that modest weight loss in even nonobese people frequently helps reduce these important risk factors". On the other hand, consider a man with a hydrostatically estimated body fat of 22%. This man has a total cholesterol of 175 $mg \cdot dl^{-1}$, an HDL-cholesterol of 55 $mg \cdot dl^{-1}$, is a nonsmoker, has a blood pressure of 110/70, and a fasting blood glucose of 100 $mg \cdot dl^{-1}$. This man has no history of chronic disease. He says that he has always been plump and so have his 80-year-old parents. This man does not need to be strongly encouraged to lose weight. If he expresses a desire for a weight loss program because he thinks it will improve his appearance, appropriate advice on exercise and dietary modification can be given.

The major point of the above examples is to encourage a more individualized approach to the interpretation of body composition values. Recognize that there is a wide range of acceptable body composition scores, not everyone is destined to be as thin as a dancer or model, and that it is probably normal to become somewhat fatter with aging.

MUSCULAR FITNESS

The term "muscular fitness" has been used to describe the integrated status of the following variables: muscular strength, muscular endurance, and flexibility. If properly conducted, programs for the development of muscular fitness can maintain or improve posture and prevent or reduce muscular low back pain. Maintenance of adequate muscular performance is also an important consideration for the promotion of the capacity of the elderly to perform essential daily tasks and to live independently.

MUSCULAR STRENGTH

Muscular strength refers to the maximal force (expressed in Newtons or kg) that can be generated by a specific muscle or muscle group. Static or isometric strength can be conveniently measured using a variety of devices, including cable tensiometers and handgrip dynamometers. Unfortunately, measures of static strength are specific both to the muscle group and joint angle involved in testing and, therefore, their utility or extrapolation to describe overall muscular strength is limited. Peak force development in such tests is commonly referred to as a "maximum voluntary contraction (MVC)".

When testing involves movement of the body or an external load, then "dynamic" or "isotonic" strength is being evaluated. Simple tests of this kind include minimal fitness tests such as the ability to perform a single push-up, pull-up, sit-up, abdominal curl or extension. Isotonic strength can also be measured using various one-repetition maximum (1RM) weight lifting tests. Valid measures of general upper body strength include the 1RM bench press and military press tests.[29] Corresponding indices of lower body strength include the upper and lower leg press tests. After warm-up and familiarization with equipment, subjects are allowed up to five trials with appropriate rest periods between to achieve a peak 1RM performance. Note that if dynamic muscular performance tests involve maximum total work performance within a short (i.e., nonfatiguing) time frame (e.g., vertical jump), then muscular power is being evaluated. Norm tables for these strength tests are available.[23]

Isokinetic testing involves the assessment of muscle tension generated throughout an entire range of joint motion at a constant speed. Equipment which allows control of the speed of joint rotation (degrees$\cdot s^{-1}$) as well as physical adjustability to test movement around various joints (e.g., knee, hip, shoulder, elbow) is available from several commercial sources. Such devices measure peak rotational force or torque, defined as "the measured ability of a rotating element to overcome turning resistance":

$$\text{Torque} = \text{Force} \cdot \text{distance}^{-1} \text{ (Newton-meters or foot-pounds)}$$

An important drawback to such equipment is that the maximal speed of joint rotation during testing is less than that of many body movements involved in exercise performance.

MUSCULAR ENDURANCE

Muscular endurance is the ability of a muscle group to execute repeated contractions (i.e., perform work) over a period of sufficient time duration to cause muscular fatigue. When testing involves static muscle contraction, the timed ability of the subject to maintain a specific percentage of MVC is usually measured as an index of muscular endurance.

Simple field tests such as the 60-second sit-up test or the maximum number of push-ups that can be performed without rest can be used to evaluate the endurance of the upper body and abdominal muscle groups, respectively.[23,24] Methods for administration and age and sex specific percentile norms for these tests are available.[12,23,24] However, the sit-up test has been criticized because of the involvement of accessory muscles (hip flexors) in addition to the abdominal muscles themselves. Although scientific proof is lacking, low abdominal strength/endurance is commonly thought to contribute to the etiology of muscular low back pain.

Weight training and "isokinetic" equipment can also be adapted to measure muscular endurance by selecting an appropriate submaximal level of resistance and time limit which will result in muscular fatigue. For example, the bench press test involves performance of standardized repetitions at a rate of 60 reps·min^{-1}. Men are tested using an 80-pound barbell and women with a 35-pound barbell. Subjects are scored by the number of successful repetitions.[24]

Tests of muscular strength and endurance must be strictly standarized in order to provide valid results. In this regard, movements used in testing must be specific to the muscle group being tested, proper movement mechanics must be utilized and subjects must be highly motivated.

FLEXIBILITY

Flexibility is the maximum ability to move a joint through a range of motion. It depends on a number of specific variables, including distensibility of the joint capsule, muscle temperature, muscle viscosity, flexibility of ligaments, etc. Like muscular strength, flexibility is specific. Therefore, no single test can be generalized to evaluate total body flexibility. The assessment of flexibility has been reviewed.[17]

Laboratory tests usually quantify flexibility in terms of range of motion, expressed in degrees. Common devices for this purpose include various goniometers, electrogoniometers, and the Leighton flexometer.[36] Field tests used for the evaluation of flexibility include the shoulder elevation test, ankle flexibility test, trunk flexion (sit-and-reach) test, and trunk extension test.

The trunk flexion or sit-and-reach test is often employed in health-oriented fitness evaluation to evaluate low back/hamstring flexibility. Poor lower back/hamstring muscle flexibility may, in conjunction with poor abdominal strength/endurance or other etiologic factors, contribute to development of muscular low back pain. However, this hypothesis remains to be substantiated from a scientific perspective. Methods to administer this test and norms based on large population percentile data are available as part of the Canadian Standardized Test of Fitness.[12] Other norm tables are also available.[23,24]

PHYSICAL FITNESS TESTING IN CHILDREN

Measurement of physical fitness in children is a common practice in school-based physical education programs. Such testing also has been employed in public health surveys,[42,43] recreational programs and, to a limited extent, in clinical settings. Fitness testing of children has a long history and traditional methods tended to emphasize measurement of motor performance components such as speed and anaerobic power. However, in recent years the measurement of health related fitness, as defined earlier in this chapter, has become a prevalent approach in children as well as adults. This change has been endorsed by the American College of Sports Medicine which has recommended that youth fitness tests emphasize health-related measures and that criterion-referenced standards be applied in interpreting the results of these tests.[2]

A detailed discussion of accepted methods of fitness testing in children is beyond the scope of this chapter. In general, the procedures recommended are similar to those described above for adults. Since most fitness testing of children occurs in field settings, inexpensive measures that are practical for use with large groups are typically employed. A survey of the current nationally promoted physical fitness test batteries for children indicates that the test items listed below are in wide use.[39,44]

Test Battery	**References**
Cardiorespiratory Endurance	
Mile run/walk for time	1,14,20,41,42,43
One-half mile run/walk (ages 6 to 7)	43
Steady state jog	3
Body Composition	
Sum of skinfold thicknesses	1,2,20,42,43
Body Mass Index	1,20,42,43
Muscular Strength/Endurance	
Pull-ups	1,20,42
Flexed arm hang	14,20,41
Modified pull-up	42
Bent-knee sit-ups or curl-ups	1,3,14,20,41,42,43
Push-ups, isometric or modified	14
Flexibility	
Sit-and-Reach test	1,3,20,42,43
V-Sit Reach	14,41

For detailed descriptions of specific test items, the reader is referred to the references cited above.

REFERENCES

1. AAHPERD: *The AAHPERD Physical Best Program.* Reston, VA: American Alliance for Health, Physical Education, Recreation and Dance, 1988.

2. American College of Sports Medicine: Opinion statement on physical fitness in children and youth. *Med Sci Sports Exerc 20*:422–423, 1988.
3. American Health and Fitness Foundation: *Fit Youth Today.* Austin, TX: American Health and Fitness Foundations, 1986.
4. Åstrand I: Aerobic work capacity in men and women with special reference to age. *Acta Physiol Scand 49*(suppl. 169):45–60, 1960.
5. Åstrand P-O and Rhyming I: A nomogram for calculation of aerobic capacity (physical fitness) from pulse rate during submaximal work. *J Appl Physiol 7*:218, 1954.
6. Balke B: A simple field test for the assessment of physical fitness. Report 63–6. Oklahoma City: Civic Aeronautic Research Institute, Federal Aviation Agency, 1963.
7. Boone T: Surface anatomy for exercise programming. In *Resource Manual for Guidelines for Exercise Testing and Prescription.* Edited by American College of Sports Medicine. Philadelphia: Lea & Febiger, 1988.
8. Bray GA and Gray DS: Obesity. Part 1—Pathogenesis. *Western J Med 149*:429–441, 1988.
9. Brozek J, Grande F, Anderson J, Keys A: Densitometric analysis of body composition: Revision of some quantitative assumptions. *Ann NY Acad Sci 110*:113–140, 1963.
10. Brozek J and Keys A: The evaluation of leanness-fatness in man: Norms and interrelationships. *Br J Nutr 5*:194–206, 1951.
11. Brozek J and Henschel A: *Techniques for Measuring Body Composition.* Washington DC: National Academy of Sciences-National Research Council, 1961.
12. *Canadian Standardized Test of Fitness (CSTF) Operations Manual,* 3rd Ed. Available from Fitness and Amateur Sport Canada, 365 Laurier Ave. West, Ottawa, Canada K1A 0X6.
13. Casperson CJ, Powell KE and Christenson GM: Physical activity, exercise and physical fitness: Definitions and distinctions for health-related research. *Public Health Reports 100*:126–131, 1985.
14. Chrysler Fund-Amateur Athletic Union: *Physical Fitness Program.* Bloomington, IN: The Chrysler Fund-Amateur Athletic Union, 1987.
15. Conway JM, Norris KH and Bodwell CE: A new approach for the estimation of body composition: Infrared interactance. *Am J Clin Nutr 40*:1123–1130, 1984.
16. Cooper KH: A means of assessing maximal oxygen intake. *JAMA 203*:201–204, 1968.
17. Corbin C: Flexibility. *Clin Sports Med 3*:101–117, 1984.
18. Fanelli MT and Kuczmarski RJ: Ultrasound as an approach to assessing body composition. *Am J Clin Nutr 39*:703–709, 1984.
19. Fitness Safety Standards Committee: *Final Report to the Minister of Tourism and Recreation on the Development of Fitness Safety Standards in Ontario (Canada).* February, 1990.
20. *Fitnessgram User's Manual.* Dallas, TX: Institute for Aerobics Research, 1987.
21. Forsyth HS and Sinning WE: The anthropometric estimation of body density and lean body weight of male athletes. *Med Sci Sports Exerc 5*:174, 1973.

22. Garrow JS: New approaches to body composition. *Am J Clin Nutr 35*:1152–1158, 1982.
23. Gettman LR: Fitness Testing. In *Resource Manual for Guidelines for Exercise Testing and Prescription.* Edited by American College of Sports Medicine. Philadelphia, Lea & Febiger, 1988.
24. Golding LA, Myers CR and Sinning WE (eds.): *Y's Way to Physical Fitness,* 3rd Ed. Champaign, IL: Human Kinetics Publishers, 1989.
25. Holly RG: Measurement of the maximal rate of oxygen uptake. In *Resource Manual for Guidelines for Exercise Testing and Prescription.* Edited by American College of Sports Medicine. Philadelphia: Lea & Febiger, 1988.
26. Howley ET and Franks BD: *Health/Fitness Instructor's Handbook.* Champaign, IL: Human Kinetics Publishers, 1986.
27. Jackson AS and Pollock ML: Generalized equations for predicting body density for men. *Br J Nutr 40*:497–504, 1978.
28. Jackson A, Pollock M and Ward A: Generalized equations for predicting body density for women. *Med Sci Sports Exerc 12*:175–182, 1980.
29. Jackson A, Watkins M and Patton R: A factor analysis of twelve selected maximal isotonic strength performances on the Universal Gym. *Med Sci Sports Exerc 12*:274–277, 1980.
30. Katch F and Katch V: The body composition profile: Techniques of measurement and applications. *Clin Sports Med 3*:31–63, 1984.
31. Keys A, Fidanza F, Karvonen M, Kimura N and Taylor H: Indices of relative weight and obesity. *J Chron Dis 254*:329–343, 1971.
32. Kline GM, Porcari JP, Hintermeister R, Freedson PS, Ward A, McCarron RF, Ross J and Rippe JM: Estimation of VO_{2max} from a one-mile track walk, gender, age, and body weight. *Med Sci Sports Exerc 19*:253–259, 1987.
33. Leighton J: An instrument and technique for the measurement of range of joint motion. *Arch Phys Med Rehabil 36*:571–578, 1955.
34. Lohman T: Skinfolds and body density and their relation to body fatness: A review. *Hum Biol 53*:181–225, 1981.
35. McArdle WD, Katch FI and Katch VL: *Exercise Physiology: Energy, Nutrition, and Human Performance,* 2nd ed. Philadelphia: Lea & Febiger, 1986.
36. Moffatt RJ: Strength and flexibility considerations for exercise prescription. In *Resource Manual for Guidelines for Exercise Testing and Prescription.* Edited by American College of Sports Medicine. Philadelphia: Lea & Febiger, 1988.
37. National Center for Health Statistics: *Health. United States, 1989.* Hyattsville, MD: Public Health Service [DHHS Publication No: (PHS) 90—1232], 1990.
38. Pate RR: The evolving definition of physical fitness. *Quest 40*:174–179, 1988.
39. Pate RR and Shephard RJ: Characteristics of physical fitness in youth. In *Perspectives in Exercise Science and Sports Medicine. Volume 2: Youth, Exercise, and Sport.* Edited by CV Gisolfi and DR Lamb. Indianapolis: Benchmark Press, Inc., 1989.
40. Pollock M, Hickman T, Kendrick Z, Jackson A, Linnerud A and Dawson G: Prediction of body density in young and middle-aged men. *J Appl Physiol 40*:300–304, 1976.

41. President's Council on Physical Fitness and Sports. *The Presidential Physical Fitness Award Program.* Washington, DC: Author, 1987.
42. Ross JG and Gilbert GG: The national children and youth fitness study: A summary of findings. *JOPERD 56*:45–50, 1985.
43. Ross JG and Pate RR: The national children and youth fitness study II: A summary of findings. *JOPERD 58*:51–56, 1987.
44. Safrit MJ: The validity and reliability of fitness tests for children: A review. *Pediatric Exer Science 2*:9–28, 1990.
45. Shephard RJ: Can we identify those for whom exercise is hazardous? *Sports Medicine 1*:75–86, 1984.
46. Siri WE: Body composition from fluid spaces and density. In *Techniques For Measuring Body Composition.* Edited by J Brozek and A Henschel. Washington, DC: National Academy of Science, 1961, pp. 223–244.
47. Siri WE: Body composition from fluid spaces and density. *Univ Calif Donner Lab Med Phys Rep,* March, 1956.
48. Wilmore JH: An anthropometric estimation of body density and lean body weight in young women. *Am J Clin Nutr 23*:267–274, 1970.
49. Wilmore J: Body composition in sports and exercise: directions for future research. *Med Sci Sports Exerc 15*:21–31, 1983.
50. Wommersley J, Durnin J, Boddy K and Mahaffy M: Influence of muscular development, obesity and age on the fat-free mass of adults. *J Appl Physiol 41*:223–229, 1976.
51. Young C, Blondon J, Tensuan R and Fryer J: Body composition studies of "older" women thirty to seventy years of age. *Ann NY Acad Sci 110*:589–607, 1963.

CHAPTER 4

Guidelines for Exercise Test Administration

CLINICAL INDICATIONS AND USES OF EXERCISE TESTING

The purpose of exercise testing is to determine physiological responses to controlled exercise stress. Clinical applications may include diagnostic, functional, and therapeutic objectives. Diagnosis and prognostic evaluation of suspected or established cardiovascular disease is the most common clinical application of exercise testing. For this purpose, standard ECG stress testing or exercise testing with radionuclide perfusion or ventriculography are used. In addition, submaximal exercise testing is used increasingly to evaluate patients soon after myocardial infarction, coronary bypass, and coronary angioplasty procedures, before discharge and during subsequent recovery. Routine exercise testing to screen for coronary artery disease (CAD) in asymptomatic low-risk patients is controversial because of the limited predictive capacity for detection of disease in this population.

Functional exercise testing is used in the determination of exercise capacity and cardiopulmonary responses in healthy individuals and in a variety of patient groups who require exercise prescription or occupational activity guidelines. Patients who have undergone repair of a congenital heart defect, valvular replacement, or cardiac transplant are also candidates for functional assessment, because many such individuals have been physically restricted before surgery and require specific guidelines for exercise. Other special groups frequently evaluated for exercise capacity include patients with chronic heart failure (CHF), diabetes, chronic renal failure, and pulmonary disease.

Finally, exercise testing may also be used to optimize medical therapy with certain classes of drugs, such as antianginal agents, antihypertensive agents, chronic heart failure agents, and anti-arrhythmic agents.

This chapter is intended to present a rational approach to clinical exercise testing based on accumulated and published experience in many exercise laboratories. It should be emphasized that these guidelines may be modified according to individual patient needs or local circumstances.[1]

MEDICAL EVALUATION PRIOR TO TESTING

The extent of medical evaluation prior to testing will depend on the risk category of the individual (apparently healthy, higher risk, or with established cardiac disease) as outlined in Chapter 1. There are three major components of the medical evaluation prior to exercise testing: medical history, physical examination, and laboratory tests.

MEDICAL HISTORY

This is usually the most important part of the pre-exercise test evaluation. Individuals should be questioned about a past or present history of the following:

- Heart attack, coronary angioplasty, or cardiac surgery
- Chest discomfort, especially with exercise
- Lightheadedness or fainting with exercise
- Shortness of breath with exercise
- Rapid heart beats or palpitations
- Heart murmurs, clicks, or unusual cardiac findings
- High blood pressure
- Stroke
- Ankle swelling
- Peripheral arterial disease, claudication
- Phlebitis, emboli
- Pulmonary disease including asthma, emphysema and bronchitis
- Abnormal blood lipids
- Diabetes
- Anemia
- Emotional disorders
- Recent illness, hospitalization or surgical procedure
- Medications of all types
- Drug allergies
- Orthopedic problems, arthritis

Family history of:
- Coronary disease
- Sudden death
- Lipid abnormalities

Other habits:
- Caffeine use
- Alcohol use
- Tobacco use
- Eating disorders

Exercise history with information on habitual level of activity: type of exercise, frequency, duration, and intensity.

PHYSICAL EXAMINATION

An abbreviated cardiovascular and pulmonary examination should be performed by the attending physician or qualified paramedical personnel:

1. Weight/percent body fat
2. Pulse rate and regularity
3. Blood pressure: supine, sitting, and standing
4. Auscultation of the lungs with specific attention to uniformity of breath sounds in all areas (absence of rales, wheezes, and rhonchi)
5. Palpation of the cardiac apical impulse
6. Auscultation of the heart with specific attention to murmurs, gallops, clicks, and rubs
7. Palpation and auscultation of carotid, abdominal, and femoral arteries
8. Palpation and inspection of lower extremities for edema and presence of arterial pulses
9. Absence or presence of xanthoma and xanthelasma
10. Orthopedic or other medical conditions which would limit exercise testing.

LABORATORY TESTS

Laboratory data are important in the determination of whether an individual fits in the higher risk category but are not absolutely necessary for safe conduct of an exercise test if history and physical examination findings are satisfactory. The following tests are useful in assessing risk and in assigning individuals to the categories described:

A. Apparently healthy or higher risk individual
   1. Total cholesterol, HDL cholesterol, and triglyceride
   2. Fasting blood glucose

B. Coronary disease
   1. Above tests plus results of all pertinent previous cardiovascular laboratory tests (i.e., resting 12-lead ECG, coronary angiography, radionuclide or echocardiography studies, previous exercise tests)
   2. Chest x ray

C. Pulmonary disease
   1. Chest x ray
   2. Routine spirometry to include vital capacity and forced expiratory flow volumes
   3. Results of other specialized pulmonary studies

CONTRAINDICATIONS TO TESTING

There are certain individuals for whom the risks of testing outweigh the potential benefits. It is important in these circumstances for the test administrator to weigh carefully the anticipated benefits and determine that these outweigh the risks. Table 4–1 outlines absolute and relative contraindications for exercise testing. Exercise testing should not be performed by patients with absolute contraindications until these conditions are stabilized. Patients with relative contraindications may be tested only after careful evaluation of potential complications.

It should be emphasized that some absolute and relative contraindications may not apply in clinical situations where an individual patient is being tested for specific reasons after a myocardial infarction (MI) or surgical procedure or to determine the need or benefit of drug therapy. Guidelines for testing in these circumstances are outlined in the subsequent section.

Several conditions preclude *reliable* diagnostic ECG information from exercise testing. These include:

1. Left bundle branch block
2. Wolff-Parkinson-White (WPW)
3. Physiological rate adaptive pacing
4. Left ventricular hypertrophy with ST changes
5. Extensive anterior wall infarction

In the presence of these conditions, exercise testing may still provide useful information on exercise capacity and hemodynamic responses to exercise.

GENERAL PRINCIPLES OF EXERCISE TESTING

Theoretically, exercise tests could be carried out with any form of exercise. Early exercise tests were conducted by having

Table 4–1. Contraindications to Exercise Testing.

Absolute Contraindications

1. A recent significant change in the resting ECG suggesting infarction or other acute cardiac events
2. Recent complicated myocardial infarction
3. Unstable angina
4. Uncontrolled ventricular dysrhythmia
5. Uncontrolled atrial dysrhythmia that compromises cardiac function
6. Third-degree A-V block
7. Acute congestive heart failure
8. Severe aortic stenosis
9. Suspected or known dissecting aneurysm
10. Active or suspected myocarditis or pericarditis
11. Thrombophlebitis or intracardiac thrombi
12. Recent systemic or pulmonary embolus
13. Acute infection
14. Significant emotional distress (psychosis)

Relative Contraindications

1. Resting diastolic blood pressure > 120 mm Hg or resting systolic blood pressure > 200 mm Hg
2. Moderate valvular heart disease
3. Known electrolyte abnormalities (hypokalemia, hypomagnesemia)
4. Fixed-rate pacemaker (rarely used)
5. Frequent or complex ventricular ectopy
6. Ventricular aneurysm
7. Cardiomyopathy, including hypertrophic cardiomyopathy
8. Uncontrolled metabolic disease (e.g., diabetes, thyrotoxicosis, or myxedema)
9. Chronic infectious disease (e.g., mononucleosis, hepatitis, AIDS)
10. Neuromuscular, musculoskeletal, or rheumatoid disorders that are exacerbated by exercise
11. Advanced or complicated pregnancy

an individual walk up and down steps at a specified rate for a prescribed duration after which a 12-lead ECG was taken. The 2 major modes of exercise testing today are treadmill walking and stationary cycling. In addition, testing with an arm ergometer may be appropriate in patients who are unable to perform leg exercise or in whom the responses to arm exercise are of interest for diagnosis of symptoms or determination of occupational work capacity.

No matter what type of equipment is used, the following principles apply to all exercise testing:

1. If there is any doubt as to the benefit of testing or the safety of testing, the test should not be performed at that time.
2. The test protocol should be selected to accommodate the individual patient's ability to perform treadmill exercise

(walking pace, anticipated exercise capacity) or cycle ergometer exercise.

3. The exercise test should begin at a MET level intensity considerably below the anticipated limitation or maximal capacity and increase gradually in 2- or 3-minute stages, with observations made at each different stage. The increase in intensity at each stage may be as large as 2 to 3 METs in healthy populations or as small as 1/2 MET in those with disease.
4. Heart rate, blood pressure, rating of perceived exertion (RPE), and patient appearance and symptoms should be monitored regularly. Grading scales for severity of angina in cardiac patients and dyspnea in pulmonary patients are especially valuable.
5. Contraindications for testing and indications for stopping exercise should be closely observed.
6. All observations should be continued for at least 4 minutes of recovery unless abnormal responses occur which would require a longer post-test observation.
7. The testing area should be 22°C (72°F) or less and the humidity 60% or less if possible.

TREADMILL TEST PROTOCOLS

Various graded treadmill exercise test protocols have been used successfully during the last decade. Several common treadmill protocols are summarized in Table 4–2.

The Bruce protocol is the most widely used treadmill protocol.[5] It involves a change in speed and grade every 3 minutes, so that the incremental increases of exercise intensity are relatively large for each stage (2 to 3 METs). The major advantage of the Bruce protocol is relative brevity. Most nonconditioned persons can complete only stage III (9 minutes). The Bruce protocol is not recommended for cardiac patients with low anginal thresholds, elderly or deconditioned patients or for post-myocardial infarction pre-discharge exercise testing. In several recent studies, researchers have shown 10 to 20% error in estimating $\dot{V}O_2$ from the Bruce protocol. This error is attributed to rapid increases in treadmill speed and grade that exceed the $\dot{V}O_2$ uptake kinetics of most cardiac patients. In addition, the Bruce protocol usually requires extensive use of handrails for support, which also contributes to error in $\dot{V}O_2$ estimates.

The Balke-Naughton treadmill protocol format utilizes con-

Table 4–2. Commonly Used Treadmill Protocols Showing Format of Speed, Grade and Minutes of Testing. MET Values are Indicated for Each Stage or Minute Interval Completed.

BRUCE PROTOCOL

Stage	*MPH*	*Grade*	*Min*	*MET Requirement** *Men*	*Women*	*Cardiac*
			1	3.2	3.1	3.6
I	1.7	10%	2	4.0	3.9	4.3
			3	4.9	4.7	4.9
			4	5.7	5.4	5.6
II	2.5	12%	5	6.6	6.2	6.2
			6	7.4	7.0	7.0
			7	8.3	8.0	7.6
III	3.4	14%	8	9.1	8.6	8.3
			9	10.0	9.4	9.0
			10	10.7	10.1	9.7
IV	4.2	16%	11	11.6	10.9	10.4
			12	12.5	11.7	11.0
			13	13.3	12.5	11.7
V	5.0	18%	14	14.1	13.2	12.3
			15	15.0	14.1	13.0

*MET values are for each minute *completed.* Note that women and cardiac patients achieve *lower* $\dot{V}O_2$ for equivalent work load. Holding on to front rail will *increase* the apparent MET capacity.

NAUGHTON-BALKE PROTOCOL

MPH	*% Grade*	*Min.*	*METS*
3.0 (Constant)	2.5	2	4.3
	5.0	2	5.4
	7.5	2	6.4
	10.0	2	7.4
	12.5	2	8.4
	15.0	2	9.5
	17.5	2	10.5
	20.0	2	11.6
	22.5	2	12.6

MODIFIED BALKE PROTOCOL

MPH	*% Grade*	*Min.*	*METS*
2.0	0	3	2.5
2.0	3.5	3	3.5
2.0	7.0	3	4.5
2.0	10.5	3	5.4
2.0	14.0	3	6.4
2.0	17.5	3	7.4
3.0	12.5	3	8.5
3.0	15.0	3	9.5
3.0	17.5	3	10.5
3.0	20.0	3	11.6
3.0	22.5	3	12.6

stant walking speeds of 2.0 to 3.3 mph with increasing grade increments (2 to 3%) every 2 or 3 minutes. The modified Balke-type protocol is more applicable to exercise testing in cardiac patients with potentially limited exercise capacities because the incremental increase in exercise intensity at each stage is more gradual and there is less chance for error in estimating $\dot{V}O_2$. Low-level predischarge exercise tests may also utilize a similar "branching" format, which can accommodate a variety of individual walking speeds. An example of a branching protocol is shown in Table 4–3. This protocol allows initial selection of an appropriate and comfortable individual walking speed (2.0 to 3.5 mph; using 0.25 mph increments). The exercise intensity is then raised by increasing the grade to attain 1 MET increments every 2 minutes. Correlation between estimated and measured $\dot{V}O_2$ is excellent (r = 0.98) for normal and post-myocardial infarction patients.[19]

CYCLE ERGOMETER TESTING

Cycle ergometer exercise testing is a useful alternative to treadmill protocols. Many patients who have difficulty with treadmill walking due to ambulatory instability or orthopedic limitations can often complete a cycle ergometer exercise test. The gradation of work intensity is easy to control, and there is

Table 4–3. Branching Treadmill Protocol.

Exercise Intensity (METs)	*Treadmill Speed (mph)* at % Grade*						
	2.0	*2.25*	*2.5*	*2.75*	*3.0*	*3.25*	*3.5*
2	0	0					
3	1.5	1	0	0	0	0	0
4	5	4	3	2	1.5	1	0.5
5	9	7	6	5	4	3	2.5
6	12.5	10	9	7.5	6.5	5.5	5
7	16	13.5	12	10	9	7.5	7
8	20	17.5	15	13	11	10	9
9		20	17.5	15	13.5	12	11
10			20	18	16	14	13
11				21	18	16.5	15
12					21	19	17

*Treadmill speed is initially selected at 0% grade to produce a brisk walking pace (2 to 3 mph) compatible with each patient's gait. Treadmill speed may be subsequently increased or decreased in branching increments of 0.25 mph (within the range of 2.0 to 3.5 mph) to maintain optimum walking speed. The percent of grade in the corresponding speed column is increased every 2 minutes to produce 1 MET increments in work intensity.

less interference with ECG and blood pressure recordings due to body motion.

Cycle ergometer protocols should begin with a "no-load" 2 minute warm-up phase, followed by progressive increases of 150 to 300 kg-m·min^{-1} (25 to 50 watts) every 2 minutes. Heart rate and blood pressure are obtained every minute, and an ECG tracing at the end of each 2-minute stage.

Most studies have shown that the peak values for heart rate during upright cycle ergometry are similar to treadmill exercise. However, $\dot{V}O_{2max}$ is 5 to 10% lower and systolic blood pressure is somewhat higher, probably due to the more limited muscle mass utilized and the gradual contribution of isometric hand grips required to stabilize the torso. Diastolic blood pressure values also tend to increase slightly, due to the isometric pressor reflex.

ARM EXERCISE TESTING

Patients with peripheral vascular disease or musculoskeletal disorders who are unable to perform treadmill or cycle ergometer exercise may be evaluated with arm exercise testing. Arm or upper extremity exercise is performed with an arm crank ergometer while the subject is seated or standing. (Standing usually permits a greater use of torso and postural muscle groups to achieve higher peak cardiopulmonary stress). Arm exercise protocols may be continuous, increasing by 25 watt (150 kg-m·min^{-1}) increments every 2 minutes, or discontinuous with stages of 25 watts for 2 minutes separated by 1 or 2 minutes of rest. Discontinuous stages are better tolerated by most patients and also permit more frequent measurement of immediate post-exercise blood pressure. It should be noted that blood pressure declines rapidly immediately after termination of upright arm cranking exercise.

Maximal arm exercise $\dot{V}O_2$ is usually 60 to 70% of that determined for leg exercise $\dot{V}O_{2max}$. Typical peak values of 600 kg-m·min^{-1} are achieved by men 50 to 65 years of age. Maximal heart rates attained during arm exercise are similar to or slightly lower than those achieved during treadmill or cycle ergometer exercise. Periodic measurement of blood pressure is possible in one arm while cranking at submaximal intensities or immediately after cessation of a 2-minute stage. Maximal blood pressure levels are difficult to obtain during exercise and the immediate post-exercise values are undoubtedly reduced from peak exercise.

Some patients with peripheral vascular disease or orthopedic limitations may perform a combined arm and leg exercise test using an arm and leg ergometer. These ergometers permit patients to utilize variable combinations of arm and leg exercise effort. Maximal exercise $\dot{V}O_2$ and heart rate are usually higher than those obtained using arm cranking exercise protocols.

Several studies have reported that the sensitivity of arm exercise testing for the detection of CAD is significantly less than treadmill exercise.[3]

RADIONUCLEAR EXERCISE TESTING

Radionuclear perfusion scintigraphy exercise testing utilizes standard treadmill or cycle ergometer protocols with ECG and blood pressure monitoring previously described. Prior to the test an intravenous catheter is inserted into an antecubital or hand vein. Radionuclide agents (e.g., ^{201}thallium) are rapidly injected at near maximal exercise (RPE 15 to 16, heart rate $\geq$ 85% max). However, it is essential to continue exercise for approximately 60 seconds following injection of the radionuclide so that initial coronary perfusion occurs at near maximal cardiac work demands. Scintigraphic imaging is obtained immediately post-exercise and after 4 hours of recovery.

Radionuclide ventriculography is performed during steady state supine or upright cycle ergometry exercise. Equilibrium ventricular angiography utilizes ^{99}technetium to label erythrocytes (blood pool) prior to exercise. First-pass ventriculography utilizes rapid injection of ^{99}technetium during peak exercise. Both methods determine resting and peak left ventricular ejection fraction. The equilibrium method allows serial measurement of left ventricular ejection fraction at submaximal and maximal exercise.

CALCULATION OF EXERCISE CAPACITY

The exercise intensity achieved on a standard maximal treadmill or cycle ergometer exercise test is a useful estimate of $\dot{V}O_{2max}$ unless abnormal responses force premature cessation of exercise. The equations and tables in Appendix D can be used to calculate the oxygen requirement for the exercise intensity achieved during an exercise test. Figure 4–1 also allows estimation of $\dot{V}O_{2max}$ and exercise capacity in METs from treadmill

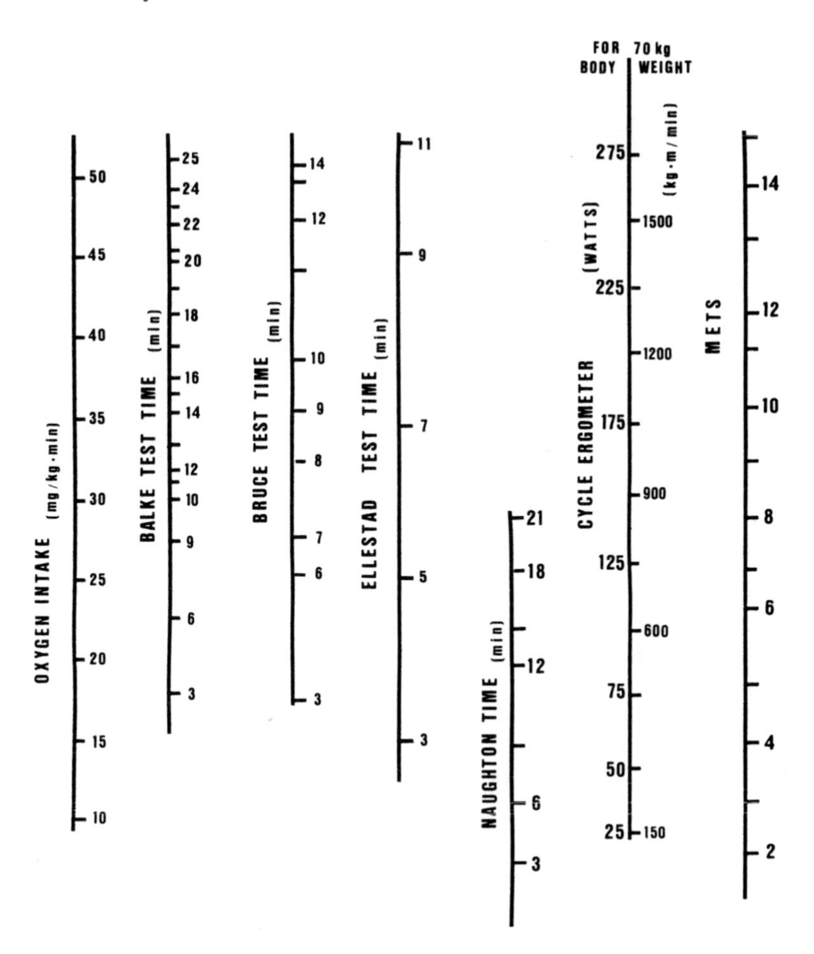

FIGURE 4–1. Estimate exercise intensity equivalents by drawing a horizontal line from the time on a given treadmill or cycle ergometer protocol to oxygen uptake (left) or MET level (right). (Modified from Pollock ML et al.: *Am Heart J 92*:39–46, 1976.)

time or cycle ergometer exercise intensity. Direct measurement of $\dot{V}O_{2max}$ is usually unnecessary for most diagnostic exercise testing. However, direct $\dot{V}O_2$ measurements are often helpful for evaluation of patients with chronic heart failure because estimated $\dot{V}O_2$ is frequently in error in this population.[24]

PATIENT INSTRUCTIONS

Patients should abstain from food, tobacco, alcohol, and caffeine for at least 3 hours prior to testing. Clothing should permit freedom of movement and include comfortable walking/running shoes. Women should bring a loose-fitting blouse with short sleeves that buttons down the front and should avoid restrictive undergarments.

For initial diagnostic exercise testing, it is helpful to have the patient discontinue prescribed cardiovascular medications if there are no anticipated adverse effects from doing so and if the referring physician agrees. All currently prescribed classes of antianginal agents will alter the hemodynamic responses to exercise and significantly reduce the sensitivity of ECG changes for ischemia. Patients who are on intermediate or high dose beta blocking agents should taper their medication over a 2- to 4-day period to minimize hyperadrenergic withdrawal responses.

INFORMED CONSENT

Individuals should sign an informed consent form prior to exercise testing. A sample consent form is included in Appendix A. The purpose of the consent form is to make certain the patient is aware of the small, but real risk of exercise testing. This risk, according to present data, is approximately 0.5 deaths per 10,000 tests in large, varied populations (see Chapter 1). The consent form should include a statement that the patient has been given an opportunity to ask questions about the procedure and has sufficient information to give the informed consent. If the subject to be tested is a minor, a legal guardian or parent must sign the consent form.

PREPARATION FOR ECG MONITORING

Electrocardiographic monitoring is an essential component of diagnostic and functional exercise testing. In most exercise ECG recording systems, a modified 10-electrode (Mason-Likar) configuration is used that permits continuous oscilloscope monitoring and recording of various combinations of the 6 standard limb and 6 precordial leads (Fig. 4–2). Studies show increased sensitivity for detection of ischemic ECG changes when multiple leads (12-lead or multiple bipolar) are employed in exercise testing. Bipolar leads in single or multiple combination (CM5, CC5) are less sensitive for diagnostic testing but are still useful and are less expensive for routine ECG monitoring in functional exercise tests.

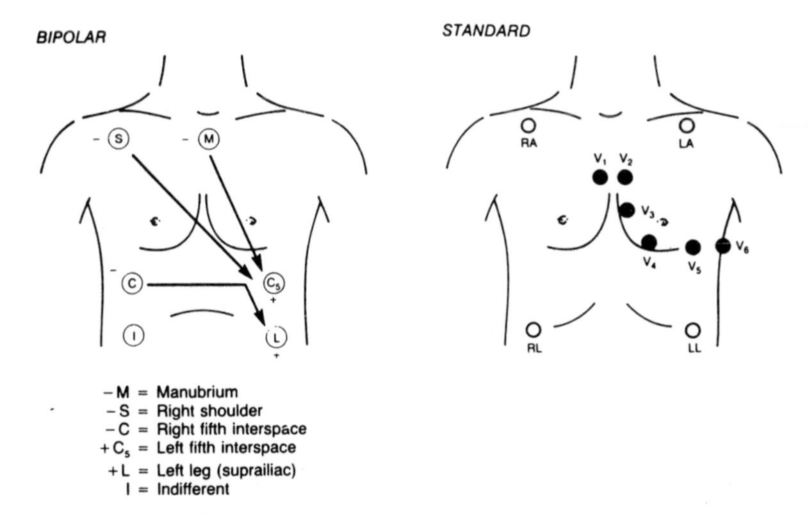

FIGURE 4–2. Electrocardiographic (ECG) leads used in exercise testing. Bipolar ECG configurations (left) are variations of V_5, using sternal (CS-5) or manubrial (CM-5) lead placements along with an indifferent reference lead. The 10-electrode (Mason-Likar) placement (right) permits standard 12-lead ECG tracings during exercise. (Modified from Chaitman B et al.: *Am J Cardiol 47*:1335–1349, 1981.)

Several recent reports have shown that the commonly used torso positioned exercise ECG lead configuration produces significant distortion of the supine baseline 12-lead resting ECG obtained using conventional extremity electrode placement. Therefore, resting 12-lead ECGs obtained in the standing or seated position prior to exercise testing may differ in frontal plane axis (more vertical) and in QRS wave forms (gain or loss of Q-waves and R-wave amplitude).

The most important determinant of satisfactory ECG monitoring is adequate preparation of skin sites for electrode placement. Skin sites must be abraded with fine sandpaper (or commercially available pads) and alcohol to remove surface epidermis and oil. After placement, each electrode should be tapped with a finger tip while the corresponding lead is monitored on the oscilloscope. Noisy leads should be readjusted or replaced.

CONDUCTING THE TEST

PATIENT INSTRUCTIONS

The protocol and sequence of the test should be explained in detail. Many patients are highly anxious before exercise testing and may perform awkwardly, with rigid walking posture and tense gripping of support rails. Their anxiety can be relieved by careful explanation, which may include a demonstration of how to walk on a treadmill (including stepping on and off). Patients should be instructed to maintain a steady walking pace and to avoid turning their head or trunk, causing loss of balance. Excessive use of support rails for balance results in major errors (15 to 20%) in estimating $\dot{V}O_2$ from treadmill speed and grade.

For cycle ergometer exercise testing the seat height should first be adjusted so that the patient's knees remain 5 to 10% flexed at maximum pedal length. A 1-minute period of no-load pedaling at the desired rate (50 to 60 rpm) is useful to demonstrate proper cycling technique. Instructions about blood pressure measurement can also be given at this time.

TEST SEQUENCE AND MEASUREMENTS

A routine set of measurements should be obtained at rest, during exercise, and during recovery. Before exercise, ECG tracings are taken with the patient supine, after 30 seconds of seated hyperventilation and after standing. Significant changes in ST-segment, T-waves, or mean frontal axis may occur after hyperventilation or standing.

During exercise, the ECG is monitored continuously by oscilloscope and recordings are made at the end of each stage or more frequently for abnormal responses. Measurements of blood pressure should be taken at 1- or 2-minute intervals to allow early identification of abnormal trends (see below). Rating of perceived exertion (RPE) is a valuable guide to effort level and participants should be queried every 2 minutes (or at the end of each stage).

Recovery should include a 2- to 4-minute period of walking (2.0 to 3.0 mph at 0% grade or no-load cycling) followed by seated rest for 2 to 4 minutes or until abnormal ECG or blood responses resolve. The recovery values for heart rate and blood pressure should be stable, but not necessarily at pre-exercise levels, before discontinuation of monitoring. In some laboratories, a supine recovery protocol is used immediately after exercise. The increase in venous return in the supine position may produce additional left ventricular preload and aid in the detection of ischemic ECG changes.

BLOOD PRESSURE RECORDING

Blood pressure should be taken in the supine, sitting, and standing positions prior to exercise. During exercise, blood pressure should be measured at least every 2 minutes throughout submaximum stages and at 1-minute intervals at maximum stages. Blood pressure must be measured at 30- to 60-second intervals in the presence of hypo- or hypertensive readings. During recovery, blood pressure is usually monitored at 1- to 2-minute intervals. Blood pressure should be measured with the subject's arm relaxed and not grasping a treadmill bar or cycle handle bar. The use of an appropriate sized blood pressure cuff and a mercury manometer mounted at eye level is important to assure accurate readings.[2]

Several models of automatic monitors are available for blood pressure measurement during exercise. These monitors utilize surface microphone or oscillographic transducers to detect the onset of systolic pressure and diastolic pressure. Analysis of pressure recordings is facilitated by microcomputer circuits. Published data show reasonable correlation with simultaneous auscultatory and intra-arterial pressures. However, in practice motion artifact frequently limits the use of automatic blood pressure monitors, especially at higher intensity exercise.

RATING OF PERCEIVED EXERTION (RPE)

Maximal heart rate varies greatly among individuals during exercise testing. Therefore, it is helpful to be able to evaluate ratings of perceived exertion to assess whether or not a test is truly maximal and to assess when maximum exercise is being approached. This may be even more important if patients are taking medications that restrict heart rate response to exercise. The perceived exertion scales illustrated in Figure 4–3 provide methods to quantify subjective exercise intensity. RPE from the category scale correlates closely with several exercise variables, including percent $\dot{V}O_{2peak}$, percent heart rate reserve, minute ventilation, and blood lactate levels. In normal individuals, heart rate will approximate RPE $\times$ 10 + 20 to 30 beats$\cdot$min^{-1} for RPEs of 11 to 16 and heart rates of 130 to 160, values in the

Category RPE Scale		Category-Ratio RPE Scale	
6		0	Nothing at all
7	Very, very light	0.5	Very, very weak
8		1	Very weak
9	Very light	2	Weak
10		3	Moderate
11	Fairly light	4	Somewhat strong
12		5	Strong
13	Somewhat hard	6	
14		7	Very strong
15	Hard	8	
16		9	
17	Very hard	10	Very, very strong
18		•	Maximal
19	Very, very hard		
20			

FIGURE 4–3. RPE scales. Original scale (6 to 20) on left and revised scale (1 to 10) on right. (From Borg GA: *Med Sci Sports Exerc 14*:377–387, 1982.)

typical intensity range for training. RPEs from 11 to 16 will also approximate a relative exercise intensity ranging from 50 to 75% of maximal METs. Numerous clinical studies have demonstrated that the category RPE scale is a reproducible measure of exertion within a wide variety of individuals regardless of age, gender, or cultural origin. The validity of RPE for estimating relative exercise intensity is also unaffected by beta blockade.

During most exercise testing, the category RPE scale is an accurate gauge of impending fatigue. Most individuals rate the ventilatory threshold (60 to 75% $\dot{V}O_{2peak}$) as somewhat hard or hard (RPE 13 to 16) and reach the subjective limit of fatigue at an RPE of 18 to 19 (very, very hard).[4] However, clinical experience indicates that 5 to 10% of persons unfamiliar with the scale tend to underestimate or suppress RPE below expected levels during the early and middle stages of testing. Three learning trials appear sufficient to reduce most errors of rating and will permit RPE to also be used as an adjunct to heart rate for monitoring exercise intensity. Test clinicians should attempt to provide a nonjudgmental and supportive atmosphere to minimize respondents' concerns over evaluation.

RPE using the category scale grows linearly as exercise intensity increases and is most closely correlated with physiological responses that also increase linearly with increasing exercise intensity such as heart rate, minute ventilation, and oxygen consumption. Category ratings work well for most exercise testing purposes. For some applications, however, it may be desirable to use Borg's newer category scale with ratio properties. True psychophysical responses to intensity stimuli appear to increase as a power function rather than a linear or log response. In other words, at both low and high intensities of exertion, subjects may need an opportunity to pick scale numbers that provide a more finely tuned subjective response to small increases in objective exercise intensity. For example, the newer category-ratio RPE scale is valid for assessing angina and it should better approximate changes in blood lactate, ventilatory equivalent for oxygen, and hormonal responses that increase exponentially during intense exercise. When using the category-ratio scale it is important that respondents clearly understand that a rating of 10 is not truly maximal. If the subjective intensity rises above a rating of 10, the person is then free to choose any larger number in proportion to 10 that describes the proportionate growth of the sensation. For example, if an increase in exercise intensity feels 20% harder than it did at the rating of 10, the RPE would be 12. If it feels 50% harder than at the rating of 10, the RPE would be 15.

To reduce problems of misinterpretation of RPE for clients and patients, it is important to use standardized instructions. Customized instructions may be needed for special applications of RPE, but the following are recommended for graded testing:

During the graded exercise test we want you to pay close attention to how hard you *feel* the work rate is. This feeling should be your total amount of exertion and fatigue, combining all sensations and feelings of physical stress, effort, and fatigue. Don't concern yourself with any one factor such as leg pain, shortness of breath or exercise intensity, but try to concentrate on your *total, inner* feeling of exertion. Don't underestimate or overestimate, just be as accurate as you can.

INTERPRETATION OF THE EXERCISE TEST

TEST END-POINTS

Normal end-points for termination of an exercise test include symptoms of muscle fatigue, hyperpnea, achievement of maximal predicted heart rate, and RPE greater than 17 (very hard). Because these responses may converge rapidly over a short period (60 to 90 seconds), careful observation and monitoring are necessary to avoid excessive stress.

Abnormal responses to exercise may require discontinuation of stress testing before attaining maximal levels of effort (Table 4–4). Important clinical criteria for immediate termination of the test include angina, dyspnea, dizziness, falling systolic blood pressure, or other indications of severe ischemia with left ventricular failure. Dangerous dysrhythmias (increasing or multiform premature ventricular contractions, ventricular tachycardia, supraventricular tachycardia, new atrial fibrillation, or A-V block) demand immediate termination of the test.

Some non-emergent abnormal responses may be evaluated on an individual basis to determine the relative risk of continuing exercise. In some instances, the goal of the test may be to establish efficacy of treatment with antianginal or antiarrhythmic drugs so that continuation of the test may be warranted.

ABNORMAL SYMPTOMS

Angina, dyspnea, and fatigue are the most common cardiac symptoms produced by exercise testing. Subjective ratings of the intensity of angina or dyspnea are graded on a scale of 1 to 4 (Table 4–5). The onset of typical angina during exercise is an

Table 4–4. Indications for Stopping an Exercise Test.

1. Progressive angina (stop at 3+ level or earlier on a scale of 1+ to 4+) (see Table 4–5)
2. Ventricular tachycardia
3. Any significant drop (20 mm Hg) of systolic blood pressure or a failure of the systolic blood pressure to rise with an increase in exercise load
4. Lightheadedness, confusion, ataxia, pallor, cyanosis, nausea, or signs of severe peripheral circulatory insufficiency
5. > 4 mm horizontal or downsloping ST depression or elevation (in the absence of other indicators of ischemia)
6. Onset of second- or third-degree A-V block
7. Increasing ventricular ectopy, multiform PVCs, or R on T PVCs
8. Excessive rise in blood pressure: systolic pressure > 250 mm Hg; diastolic pressure > 120 mm Hg
9. Chronotropic impairment
10. Sustained supraventricular tachycardia
11. Exercise-induced left bundle branch block
12. Subject requests to stop
13. Failure of the monitoring system

Table 4–5. Angina and Dyspnea Scales.

Angina Scale	
1+	Light, barely noticeable
2+	Moderate, bothersome
3+	Severe, very uncomfortable
4+	Most severe pain ever experienced
Dyspnea Scale	
+1	Mild, noticeable to patient but not observer
+2	Mild, some difficulty, noticeable to observer
+3	Moderate difficulty, but can continue
+4	Severe difficulty, patient cannot continue

accurate predictor of CAD; however, fewer than 50% of patients with CAD experience angina with maximal effort exercise. In addition, the degree of anginal symptoms is poorly correlated with the extent of disease. The onset of angina, dyspnea, or fatigue at low exercise loads (3 to 4 METs), however, is usually predictive of multiple vessel CAD and poor cardiac function.

Mild (grade 1) angina or atypical chest pain does not require immediate termination of the exercise test. The patient may be observed while continuing the exercise test for short periods if ECG findings and blood pressure levels stabilize. A trial administration of sublingual nitroglycerin is a useful diagnostic challenge that may confirm the presence of angina in the absence of characteristic ECG findings.

Dyspnea may be a dominant exercise symptom in severe stenosis of the left main coronary or anterior descending coronary artery. Dyspnea is usually accompanied by poor exercise capacity and impaired systolic blood pressure responses or rapidly decreasing systolic blood pressure values.

CARDIOVASCULAR RESPONSES

Increases in heart rate and blood pressure usually occur in proportion to exercise intensity. The average age-predicted maximal heart rate value may be obtained from published tables or may be estimated from regression equations (see Chapter 2). The variability of age-predicted maximal heart rates is wide ($\pm$ 10 to 15 beats·min^{-1}) and, therefore, they should not be used as an absolute end-point for termination of the exercise test.

Exercise tests that fail to elicit 85% of predicted maximal heart rate are usually considered submaximal and not a valid cardiovascular stress. Patients with cardiac disease may show a restricted heart rate increase (chronotropic impairment) in response to progressive exercise.[9]

Maximal blood pressure values usually occur at peak heart rate. Normal values for maximal blood pressure may vary widely (160 to 220/50 to 90). Hypertensive blood pressure responses are usually defined as a systolic pressure greater than or equal to 225 and a diastolic pressure of 90 or above. Discontinuation of exercise testing is recommended when the systolic pressure exceeds 250 or the diastolic pressure is 120 or greater.

Hypotensive or restricted blood pressure response patterns are often noted in individuals with severe ischemic heart disease or heart failure. Hypotensive responses include: (1) an inadequate rise in systolic pressure (less than 20 mm Hg increase from rest); (2) a fall in systolic blood pressure below pre-exercise rest levels; or (3) decreasing systolic pressure (−20 mm Hg from previous stable or rising level). These responses are signs of poor ventricular function that require termination of exercise.[11] An isolated increase in diastolic pressure (+25 mm Hg above rest) during exercise is also a predictor of underlying CAD.

Exercise-induced heart rate and blood pressure changes are characteristically attenuated by beta blockade. For patients receiving therapeutic beta blockade, peak heart rate may be limited to 50 or 60% of the predicted maximal rate, with a corresponding rise in systolic pressure of only 20 to 30 mm Hg. The blood pressure responses in patients on vasodilators (hydralazine, calcium channel blockers, alpha blockers, ACE inhibitors) are variably attenuated. This effect is most pronounced in patients with impaired left ventricular function who are treated to attain afterload reduction. In these patients exercise may be surprisingly well tolerated in spite of markedly restricted blood pressure increases.

ELECTROCARDIOGRAPHIC RESPONSES

Normal and common abnormal ECG responses to exercise are illustrated in Figure 4–4. The normal pattern of exercise-induced ECG change includes rate-related shortening of the QT interval and superposition of the P- and T-waves. The amplitude of the R-wave decreases (from resting height), and the amplitudes of septal Q-waves and T-waves increase. The ST-segment shows a progressively positive upslope, beginning

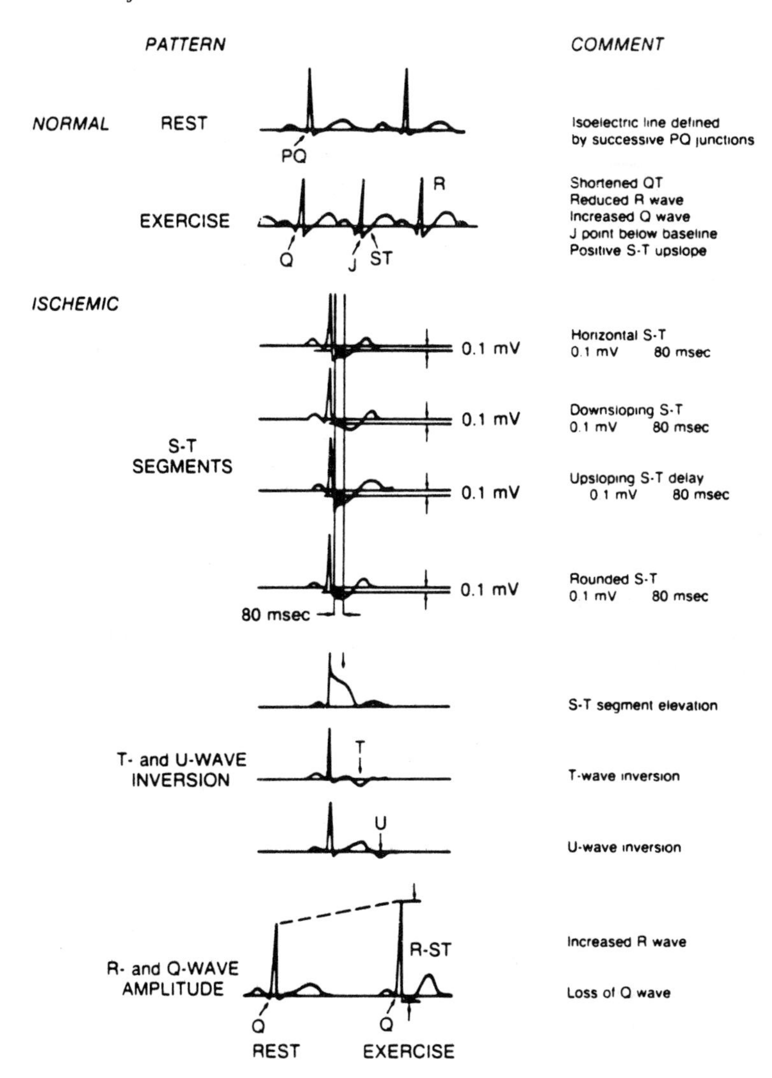

FIGURE 4–4. Common abnormal electrocardiographic (ECG) responses to exercise correlated with myocardial ischemia. See text for detailed discussion.

from the J-point (which is usually displaced below the isoelectric baseline) and returning to above the baseline within 60 to 80 milliseconds (msec). (Exercise ECG baseline is defined by successive isoelectric PQ junctions.)

ST-SEGMENT CHANGES

ST-segment depression and delayed repolarization are widely accepted diagnostic criteria for myocardial ischemia. Most authorities consider ST depression of 1.0 mm (0.1 mV) below the resting post-hyperventilation baseline for a duration of 80 msec or longer from the J-point as significant evidence of myocardial ischemia. The pattern of classic ST depression may vary from horizontal to downsloping. Rounded ST depression and delayed upsloping patterns may also occur and are equally predictive of CAD when the ST-segment remains less than 1.0 mm below baseline 80 msec after the J-point.[6,9] Interpretation of ST depression may be affected by the pre-exercise ECG configuration (left ventricular hypertrophy) and pharmacologic agents (digoxin). When ST depression is a baseline finding, an additional 1.0 mm of depression is required as evidence of ischemia.[6]

The onset, duration, and magnitude of ST depression usually correlates with the severity of myocardial ischemia. Early onset ST depression of greater than 2.0 mm that lasts 5 minutes or more into the recovery stage is strongly predictive of three-vessel or left main coronary artery stenosis. No definitive criteria are established for discontinuing exercise on the basis of asymptomatic ST depression. Some laboratories set 4 to 5 mm depression as an arbitrary value in the absence of other limiting factors.

The relationship between the magnitude of ST depression and incremental increase in heart rate (ST/HR) is a useful index of myocardial ischemia. Recent studies indicate that the ST/HR slope and the ΔST/HR index (average change of ST depression with heart rate throughout the exercise test) improve the sensitivity and specificity of ECG exercise testing for the detection of CAD.[19]

ST-segment elevation during exercise may be caused by several mechanisms. Most commonly, ST elevation is seen in leads overlying regional ventricular dyskinesia or aneurysm formation. Acute transmural ischemia may also produce ST elevation during exercise, and it is frequently associated with severe left main stem or anterior descending coronary artery stenosis.[21,24] Coronary spasm induced during exercise may produce variable patterns of ST elevation or depression.

There is no reliable relationship between the surface orientation of ECG leads that show ST depression and the anatomic localization of coronary artery stenosis. Thus, ST depression in the interior leads (2,3,avf) does not necessarily correspond to right or circumflex coronary stenosis.[22]

R-WAVE AMPLITUDE

A progressive increase in R-wave amplitude or failure of the R-wave to decrease with exercise is an ancillary finding in myocardial ischemia. The combination of increases in R-wave amplitude and ST depression is an additional index of ischemic response. Although this finding is controversial, the assessment of R-wave amplitude may be useful in the interpretation of equivocal ST depression, and is probably the only useful ECG indicator of ischemia in left bundle branch block.

T-WAVE CHANGES

Changes in T-wave polarity and amplitude may be seen during exercise stress. Unfortunately, wide variations in T-wave responses occur, even in healthy subjects. Most healthy young men have increased T-wave amplitude during and immediately after exercise. Some normal patients may show flattening and inversion of T-waves as a result of hyperventilation, hypokalemia, and superimposed exercise stress. T-wave inversion occurring in the post-exercise recovery period must be interpreted in conjunction with other test responses. Some studies have reported that normalization of inverted resting T-waves during exercise is an indicator of ischemia. However, this finding frequently occurs with simultaneous ischemic ST depression. Thus, the usefulness of T-wave changes as independent criteria for ischemia is limited.

U-WAVE INVERSION

U-wave inversion during or after exercise has been correlated with myocardial ischemia and significant stenosis of the left anterior coronary artery. The inversion pattern is defined as a discrete negative deflection within the T-P segment and is best appreciated in the V_5 (or equivalent) precordial lead. The mechanism of U-wave inversion is not known. In initial reports, researchers suggest U-wave inversion provides additional confirmation of severe or proximal left anterior descending CAD when seen in conjunction with ST depression, and may be predictive of CAD in the absence of ST depression.

DYSRHYTHMIAS

Exercise-associated dysrhythmias occur in healthy subjects as well as patients with cardiac disease. Increased sympathetic drive and changes in extracellular and intracellular electrolytes, pH, and oxygen tension contribute to disturbances in myocardial and conducting tissue automaticity and re-entry, which are major mechanisms of dysrhythmias.

SUPRAVENTRICULAR DYSRHYTHMIAS

Isolated atrial premature contractions are common and require no special precautions. Chaotic atrial rhythm, atrial flutter, or atrial fibrillation may occur in organic heart disease or secondary to endocrine, metabolic, or drug effects (hyperthyroidism, alcoholic cardiomyopathy, post-alcohol consumption "holiday heart," and digoxin toxicity).

Sustained supraventricular tachycardia (SVT) is occasionally induced by exercise and may require pharmacological treatment or electroconversion if discontinuation of exercise or use of vagal reflex maneuvers fail to abolish the rhythm. Patients who experience exercise-induced SVT may be evaluated by repeated exercise testing after appropriate treatment.

VENTRICULAR DYSRHYTHMIAS

Exercise-induced ventricular dysrhythmias are a more serious response. Isolated premature ventricular complexes or contractions (PVCs) may occur in 30 to 40% of healthy subjects and in 50 to 60% of patients with CAD during exercise. In follow-up studies, a higher rate of coronary events occurred in patients who exhibit both PVCs and ST-segment depression. In addition, results of angiographic studies show a greater degree of CAD in patients who had exercise-induced and post-exercise PVCs. PVCs may occur in association with a wide variety of underlying non-coronary disorders, including mitral valve prolapse, hypertrophic and idiopathic cardiomyopathy, and valvular heart disease.

The diagnostic significance of induction or suppression of PVC activity during exercise testing is difficult to interpret.

PVCs in healthy young adults are usually abolished with exercise. However, significant CAD may be found in patients who also show rate suppression of PVCs during exercise. The daily variability of PVC activity is considerable. Sequential exercise tests on the same day may also yield widely differing rates of PVCs.

Criteria for terminating exercise tests for ventricular ectopic beats usually include increasing frequency, multiform appearance, coupling and salvos of ventricular tachycardia. The decision to stop exercise stress may also be influenced by simultaneous evidence of ischemia or symptoms of angina.

PREDICTIVE VALUE OF EXERCISE TESTING

The predictive value of ECG exercise testing for the detection of CAD is controlled by the principles of conditional probability (Table 4–6). Three factors that determine the predictive outcome of exercise testing (and all other laboratory tests) are: *sensitivity* and *specificity* of the test procedure and the *prevalence* of the disease or condition in the population tested.

SENSITIVITY

Sensitivity is the percent of patients tested with CAD who show positive test results. Exercise ECG sensitivity for the detection of CAD is usually based on subsequent angiographic findings of coronary stenosis of 50 to 70% in at least one vessel. A true-positive ECG exercise test (ST depression of 1.0 mm for 80 msec) correctly identifies a patient with CAD. False-negative test results show nondiagnostic ECG changes and fail to identify patients with true CAD. Therefore, the sensitivity of ECG ex-

Table 4–6. Predictive Value of Exercise ECG Responses.

$$\text{Sensitivity} = \frac{TP}{TP + FN}$$

$$\text{Specificity} = \frac{TP}{TN + FP}$$

$$\begin{array}{c}\text{Predictive Value} \\ \text{(positive test)}\end{array} = \frac{TP}{TP + FP}$$

$$\begin{array}{c}\text{Predictive Value} \\ \text{(negative test)}\end{array} = \frac{TN}{TN + FN}$$

TP = True-Positive (+ Exercise Test and CAD)
FP = False-Positive (+ Exercise Test and no CAD)
TN = True-Negative (− Exercise Test and no CAD)
FN = False-Negative (− Exercise Test and CAD)

ercise testing is reduced from unity depending on the number of false-negative tests.

Common factors that contribute to false-negative results of exercise tests are summarized in Table 4–7. Test sensitivity is decreased by inadequate or submaximal stress, insufficient ECG leads, and drugs that alter cardiac work responses to exercise or reduce ischemia (beta blockers, nitrates, and calcium channel blocking agents). Pre-existing ECG changes, such as left bundle branch block or loss of precordial R-wave voltage from prior anterior infarction, limit test interpretation for ischemic ECG responses. If the criteria for a positive test are increased (from 1.0 to 2.0 mm ST depression), overall sensitivity decreases because a significant number of true-positive tests (with less than 2.0 mm ST depression) are excluded.

Sensitivity is increased by the use of maximal effort stress testing, multiple-lead ECG monitoring, computer analysis of ECG records, and additional criteria for abnormal test responses, such as low work capacity, poor blood pressure response and other ECG findings. If the criteria for a positive test are reduced (0.5 mm ST depression), the sensitivity increases but the rate of false-positive tests also increases.

SPECIFICITY

The specificity of exercise tests is determined by the percent of normal subjects (without CAD) who show a negative or nondiagnostic stress test. A true-negative test correctly identifies a person without disease. Specificity is reduced by false-positive tests in persons without CAD.

Many conditions may cause individuals to have false-positive exercise ECG responses (Table 4–8). Ischemic ST changes may occur as a result of pathophysiologic states not related to coronary artery stenosis. Left ventricular hypertrophy, anemia, hypoxia, and coronary spasm are common underlying causes of

Table 4–7. Causes of False-Negative Test Results.

1. Failure to reach an adequate exercise workload
2. Insufficient number of leads to detect ECG changes
3. Failure to use other information such as systolic blood pressure drop, symptoms, dysrhythmias, or heart rate response, in test interpretation
4. Single-vessel disease
5. Good collateral circulation
6. Musculoskeletal limitations before cardiac abnormalities occur
7. Technical or observer error

Table 4–8. Causes of False-Positive Test Results.

1. A pre-existing abnormal resting ECG (e.g., ST-T abnormalities)
2. Cardiac hypertrophy
3. Wolff-Parkinson-White syndrome and other conduction defects
4. Hypertension
5. Drugs (e.g., digitalis)
6. Cardiomyopathy
7. Hypokalemia
8. Vasoregulatory abnormalities
9. Sudden intense exercise
10. Mitral valve prolapse
11. Pericardial disorders
12. Pectus excavatum
13. Technical or observer error
14. Coronary spasm
15. Anemia
16. Female gender

false-positive responses to exercise. Abnormal ST repolarization related to digoxin therapy, pre-excitation conduction patterns, type I antiarrhythmic drugs, phenothiazines, and lithium can produce apparent ischemic ST changes in normal subjects. False-positive ECG responses occur more frequently in women (20 to 50 years of age) for undetermined reasons.

Specificity and sensitivity of exercise ECG responses have been studied in great detail. Most data show sensitivity varies from 50 to 90% and specificity varies from 60 to 98%. The wide variation in these reported values has been attributed to significant differences in patient selection, test protocols, ECG criteria for a positive test, and angiographic definition of CAD. In studies that controlled these factors, the pooled results show a sensitivity of 71% and a specificity of 73%.[9]

PREDICTIVE VALUE

The predictive value of exercise testing is a measure of how accurately a test result (positive or negative) correctly identifies the presence or absence of CAD in patients tested. The most important determinant of predictive value is the pretest likelihood of CAD in the patient, which can be estimated from published tables (Table 4–9). For example, male patients over 50 years of age with typical angina have a 90 to 95% pretest likelihood of disease; therefore, the predictive value of a positive test approaches 100%. In this case little additional information is gained by exercise testing. The pretest likelihood of disease in a 45-year-old man with atypical chest pain is reduced

Table 4–9. Prevalence of CAD According to Age, Gender, and Symptoms.

Age	Symptoms			
	None	*Non-Anginal*	*Atypical*	*Typical*
(Women)				
35	0.3	1	4	26
45	1	3	13	55
55	3	8	32	79
65	8	19	54	91
(Men)				
35	2	5	22	70
45	6	14	46	87
55	10	22	59	92
65	12	28	67	94

Values are %. Adapted from Ellested et al.: The false-positive stress test. *Am J Cardiol 40*:681–685, 1977.

Table 4–10. Predictive Value of a Positive and Negative Exercise Test (ET) According to Gender and Pretest Risk of CAD.

Clinical History	*Gender*	*Predictive Value (%)*	
		+ET	*−ET*
Typical angina	M	96	35
	F	73	67
Probable angina	M	87	56
	F	54	78
Non-anginal chest discomfort	M	39	86
	F	6	95

Adapted from Weiner et al.: *N Engl J Med 301*:230–235, 1979.

to between 40 to 50%. A positive test response would have a predictive value range of 75 to 85%. A female patient, 45 years of age with atypical chest pain, however, would have a lower pretest likelihood of disease (10 to 15%), and a positive test would have a predictive value of only 35 to 45%. Finally, young patients in the age range of 30 to 35 years with non-anginal chest pain also have a low pretest likelihood of disease (5%), and accordingly, have only a 15% predictive value for a positive test. Thus, an individual's pretest probability of having coronary disease based on age, gender, risk factors, symptoms, etc. strongly influences how one interprets an abnormal response in that individual.[13,25] Useful tables and graphs have been developed which give a quantitative estimate of this probability of disease based on the pre-test probabilities (Table 4–10) and the magnitude of ST-segment depression or elevation during the test (Fig. 4–5).

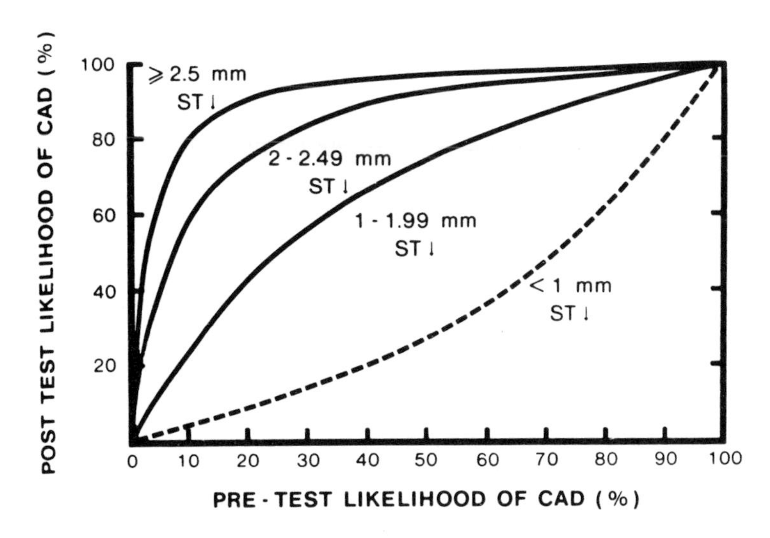

FIGURE 4–5. Relationship of pre-test vs. post-test likelihood of CAD as a function of exercise-induced ST-segment depression. Solid lines show an increasing probability of CAD with increasing ST depression. Dotted line indicates nondiagnostic or negative exercise ECG. Note that the probability of positive outcome increases exponentially with pretest likelihood regardless of ST changes. (Reprinted with permission from Epstein SE: *Am J Cardiol 46*:491–499, 1980.)

ENHANCEMENT OF PREDICTIVE VALUE

The diagnostic and prognostic accuracy of exercise test results may be improved by using additional criteria for interpretation, including quantitative description of the onset, depth, duration, and number of leads showing ST-segment depression and other ECG changes (R-wave amplitude and ventricular ectopic activity). Recent studies indicate that computer analysis of exercise ECG ST-segment depression area significantly increases the level of accuracy for detection of CAD.[17,18]

Other non-ECG criteria, such as duration of exercise or MET level attained, systolic blood pressure response pattern, maximal heart rate, rate-pressure product, and symptoms of angina or dyspnea, must be considered in the overall interpretation of exercise test results. Multivariate analysis of these variables in combination with ECG criteria show improved overall sensitivity for detection of CAD and higher specificity for the absence of multivessel CAD in patients with probable angina. Multiple exercise criteria, however, provide limited added diagnostic value to the clinical assessment of patients with atypical angina or chest pain.

One example of a prognostic treadmill score utilizes exercise time, ST displacement and angina index (0 = none, 1 = nonlimiting, 2 = limiting):

$$\text{Prognostic score} = \text{exercise time (min)} - [5 \cdot \text{ST displacement (mm)}] - [4 \cdot \text{angina index}]$$

This combination of exercise variables has been shown to accurately identify low (5 or more points), medium (−10 to +4), and high (−11 or less) risk patients.[21]

COMPARISON WITH RADIONUCLIDE IMAGING

Advances in radionuclide myocardial perfusion and ventricular angiography have greatly improved the predictive value of exercise stress testing for CAD. The reported sensitivity and specificity from both radionuclide methods are 10 to 15% greater than those of the standard exercise ECG. The combined use of radionuclide and ECG stress testing usually provides a substantial increase in sensitivity with no loss in specificity.

Exercise radionuclide studies often reveal myocardial ischemic changes at submaximal exercise intensities and heart rate before the onset of abnormal ECG responses. Therefore, adequate assessment of patients who are unable to perform near maximal exercise because of orthopedic or pulmonary limitation is possible. In addition, abnormal ECG patterns (resulting from left bundle branch block, prior anterior MI, Wolff-Parkinson-White syndrome, and digoxin use) that preclude satisfactory interpretation of exercise ECGs may be evaluated using radionuclide studies.

Radionuclide techniques are especially helpful in the evaluation of typical or atypical angina with apparently normal exercise or equivocal (discordant) ECGs and for the evaluation of probable false-positive exercise ECG responses. In these cases the results of clinical risk evaluation, exercise ST depression and radionuclide perfusion scintigraphy provide a rational incremental testing strategy for determining prognostic risk of CAD (see Fig. 4–6).[20]

For example, in a patient with intermediate CAD risk who has a positive ECG exercise test, a positive scintigraphy study

NORMAL RESTING ELECTROCARDIOGRAM
(Sequential Testing)

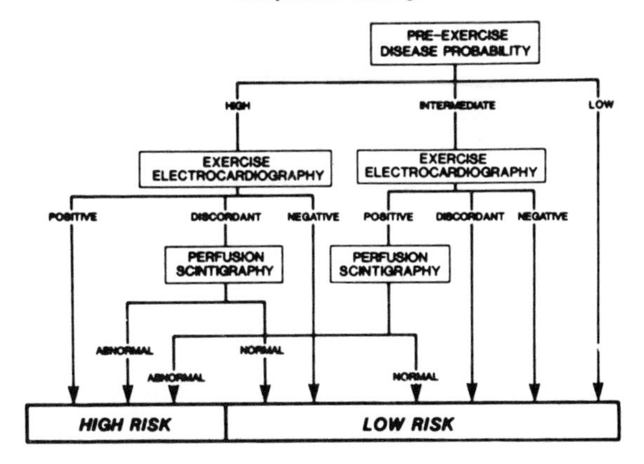

ABNORMAL RESTING ELECTROCARDIOGRAM
(Uniform Testing)

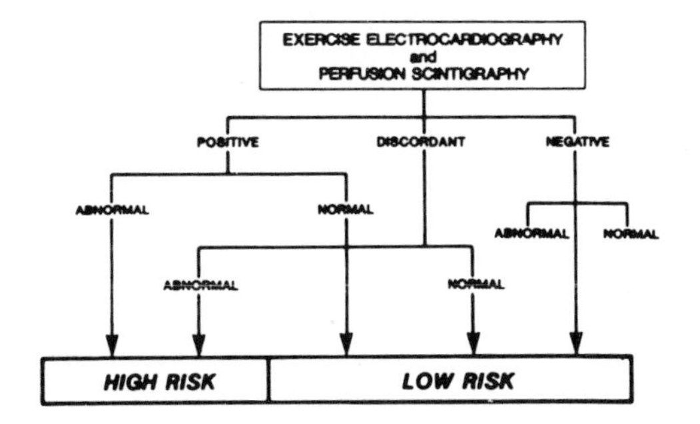

FIGURE 4–6. Incremental testing strategy for CAD risk utilizing serial results of pretest clinical risk (high, intermediate, low), exercise ECG and radionuclide perfusion scintigraphy. Top panel shows sequential testing in patients with normal baseline ECG. Bottom panel uses combined ECG and perfusion scintigraphy (uniform) testing in patients with abnormal baseline ECG. Results of these tests define low and high risk groups. (Negative ET = < 1 mm ST ↓, > 85% max heart rate; discordant ET = < 1 mm ST ↓, ≥ 85% max heart rate; positive ET = ≥ 1 mm ST ↓, < 85% max heart rate). (Reprinted with permission from Ladenheim et al.: *Am J Cardiol 59*:270–277, 1987.)

would confirm the diagnosis of CAD and an increased probability for future cardiac events (> 20%), while a negative scintigraphy test would reduce the risk to less than 5%. In another patient with a high probability of CAD risk and an equivocal (discordant) ECG exercise test, a positive exercise scintigraphy study also confirms the diagnosis of CAD and high risk of cardiac events (> 30%), while a negative scintigraphy study would reduce the probability to 5%.

FOLLOW-UP EVALUATION

Many individuals who have abnormal exercise tests with onset of ischemia at moderate or high levels of exertion may not need to have coronary angiography. These individuals can be followed with periodic exercise tests to see if the abnormalities observed increase with time. Patients with an abnormal exercise response who manifest greater abnormality on subsequent tests or the same abnormality at a lower exercise level are more likely to have progression of CAD and may require coronary angiography. Noninvasive radionuclide studies may also be done to further assess the likelihood that an abnormal exercise test is the manifestation of coronary disease.

EARLY POST-INFARCTION PRE-DISCHARGE EXERCISE TESTING

Exercise testing of patients soon after myocardial infarction or other cardiac events provides useful prognostic and therapeutic information. Low-level treadmill exercise tests usually involve the use of a constant speed (2.0 to 2.5 mph) with 1 MET increases in grade every 2 to 3 minutes (see Branching protocol, Table 4–2). Modified end-points include 75% predicted maximal heart rate (60% with beta blockade); 4 to 6 METs of treadmill or equivalent cycle ergometer work; and usual end-points for abnormal ECG, dysrhythmias, attenuated or falling systolic blood pressure, and symptoms.[8,9,15]

Results of multiple studies show that patients who develop angina, additional ST-segment depression (> 1 mm from rest), complex ventricular ectopic activity or systolic hypotension during submaximal exercise are at high risk for future reinfarction or sudden death. Coronary angiography performed in these patients reveals a high incidence of residual multivessel disease.[8]

The timing of low-level exercise testing after infarction varies widely. Predischarge exercise test studies are reported from 3 days to 3 weeks after infarction. Sequential exercise tests have shown that the ST depression noted 2 to 3 weeks after myocardial infarction was also detected at 6 to 11 weeks. Abnormal blood pressure levels, ventricular ectopic activity, and angina may resolve with the second test. An apparently normal low-level predischarge exercise test should be followed up with a symptom-limited exercise test 4- to 6-weeks post-event.

Exercise testing after myocardial infarction also provides guidelines for resumption of activities. Patients who show no abnormalities may resume normal daily activities and begin participation in supervised exercise training programs. Return to physically demanding occupations should be based on symptom-limited exercise testing. In some cases, work simulation exercise testing may be used to determine patient capacity for specific occupations.[17]

CHRONIC HEART FAILURE

Functional exercise testing is useful for evaluation and medical management of patients with chronic heart failure (CHF). Recent studies have shown that clinical classification of CHF status is most accurately determined by maximal exercise capacity (Table 4–11). Direct measurement of $\dot{V}O_{2max}$ is preferable to estimated values due to the significant effect of even a 1 MET error in patients with low exercise capacities (3 to 5 METs). Treadmill or cycle ergometer protocols with small increments of exercise intensity increases (½ to 1 MET) are recommended (Table 4–3).

CHF patients show characteristic patterns of abnormal hemodynamic responses to exercise. These include:

- impaired heart rate response
- restricted or hypotensive systolic blood pressure response
- impaired stroke volume and left ventricular ejection fraction

Table 4–11. Classification of CHF by Oxygen Uptake.

Class	*Severity of Symptoms*	$\dot{V}O_{2max}$ *(ml·kg·min⁻¹)*	*METs*
A	mild to none	> 20	> 6
B	mild to moderate	16–20	4–6
C	moderate to severe	10–16	3–4
D	severe	6–10	2–3
E	very severe	< 6	< 2

Modified from Weber et al.: *Circulation 65*:1213–1223, 1982.

- elevated systemic vascular resistance

The end-point for exercise in CHF patients is usually muscular fatigue and/or dyspnea. Peak exercise heart rate is usually well below predicted values for age. Even though $\dot{V}O_{2max}$ is markedly reduced, the onset of anaerobic (ventilatory) threshold still occurs at 75% of $\dot{V}O_{2max}$.

Exercise capacity is strongly correlated with prognosis in CHF. Patients with a $\dot{V}O_{2max}$ less than 4 METs have a poor prognosis, while patients with a $\dot{V}O_{2max}$ greater than 8 METs fall into a favorable prognostic category. The intermediate group (4 to 8 METs) show moderately reduced prognosis for survival. In this group, treatment with vasodilator agents frequently produces substantial increases in functional capacity and improvement in prognosis.

A number of studies have shown that exercise capacity in patients with CHF is independent of resting left ventricular function parameters. Patients with left ventricular ejection fractions less than 30% may perform surprisingly well during short-term exercise testing.[24]

POST-TEST PATIENT BRIEFING

Patient education following the exercise test is one of the most important, and often neglected, components of exercise testing. It is important to clearly explain to each patient the relevant findings and their significance. Care should be taken not to make an absolute diagnosis on the basis of exercise test results alone. Patients should be told about risks and likelihood of disease rather than presence or absence of disease. This period of discussion and explanation following the test is also a good time to further observe the effect of exercise on the patient. Patients should be given appropriate information on the ECG, blood pressure response, pulse rate, and fitness level. It is helpful to have a chart available to show patents their achieved fitness level and how this compares with averages and norms for patients in similar age groups. Discussion of the appropriate exercise heart rate and principles of aerobic exercise may begin at this time.

EMERGENCIES

All personnel concerned with exercise testing should be trained in basic cardiopulmonary resuscitation (CPR) and preferably Advanced Cardiac Life Support (ACLS). Telephone numbers for emergency assistance should be clearly posted on all telephones. Emergency plans should be established and posted and regular drills should be conducted at least quarterly for all personnel.

If a problem occurs during exercise testing, the physician available should be immediately summoned. The physician should make the decision whether or not to call for evacuation to the nearest hospital if testing is not carried out in the hospital. If a physician is not available and there is any question as to the status of the patient, then emergency transportation to the closest hospital should be immediately summoned. Except for defibrillation, placing an intravenous catheter, and treatment of ventricular dysrhythmias, ACLS should usually be carried out in the hospital and not in the testing station unless the physician or medical staff is experienced and competent in all aspects of ACLS. The following equipment and drugs should be available in any area where maximal exercise testing is performed:

EQUIPMENT
- Defibrillator-monitor
- Airway equipment
- Oxygen
- AMBU bag with pressure release valve
- Suction equipment
- Intravenous sets and stand
- Intravenous fluids
- Syringes and needles in multiple sizes
- Adhesive tape

DRUGS (IV form unless otherwise indicated)
- Lidocaine
- Epinephrine
- Atropine
- Isoproterenol
- Procainamide
- Sodium bicarbonate
- Bretylium
- Verapamil
- Propranolol or Esmolol
- Diazepam
- Dopamine

Nitroglycerine
Furosemide
Nitroglycerine tablets or oral spray

REFERENCES

1. American Heart Association: Guidelines for exercise testing. *Circulation 75*:653A–667A, 1986.
2. American Heart Association: Recommendations for human blood pressure determination by sphygmomanometers. Dallas: AHA, 1980.
3. Balady GJ, Weiner DA, McCabe CH and Ryan TJ: Value of arm exercise testing in detecting coronary artery disease. *Am J Cardiol 55*:37–39, 1985.
4. Borg G and Linderholm H: Perceived exertion and pulse rate during graded exercise in various age groups. *Acta Med Scand* [Suppl] *472*:194–206, 1967.
5. Bruce RA: Exercise testing for ventricular function. *N Engl J Med 296*:671–675, 1977.
6. Chaitman BR: The changing role of the exercise electrocardiogram as a diagnostic and prognostic test for chronic ischemic heart disease. *JACC 8*:1195–1210, 1986.
7. Chow RJ and Wilmore JH: The regulation of exercise intensity by ratings of perceived exertion. *J Cardiac Rehab 4*:382–387, 1984.
8. DeBusk RF, Blomqvist GC, Kouchoukos NT, Leupker RV, Miller HS, Moss AJ, Pollock ML, Reeves TJ, Selvester RH, Stason WB, Wagner GS and Willman V: Identification and treatment of low-risk patients after acute myocardial infarction and coronary-artery by-pass graft surgery. *N Engl J Med 314*:161–166, 1986.
9. Detrano R and Froelicher VF: Exercise testing: Uses and limitations considering recent studies. *Prog Cardiovasc Dis 31*:173–204, 1988.
10. Dishman RK: Behavioral barriers to health-related physical fitness. In *Epidemiology, Behavior Change, and Intervention in Chronic Disease.* Edited by LK Hall and GC Meyer. Champaign IL: Human Kinetics Publishers, 1988.
11. Dubach P, Froelicher VF, Klein J, Oakes D, Grover-McKay M and Friis R: Exercise-induced hypotension in a male population. *Circulation 78*:1380–1387, 1988.
12. Ellestad MH, Savitz S, Bergdall D and Teske J: The false-positive stress test: Multivariate analysis of 215 subjects with hemodynamic, angiographic and clinical data. *Am J Cardiol 40*:681–685, 1977.
13. Epstein SE: Implications of probability analysis on the strategy used for noninvasive detection of coronary artery disease. *Am J Cardiol 46*:491–499, 1980.
14. Guttmann MC, Squires RW, Pollock ML, Foster C and Anholm J: Perceived exertion-heart rate relationship during exercise testing and training in cardiac patients. *J Cardiac Rehab 1*:52–59, 1981.
15. Hamm LF, Stull GA and Crow RS: Exercise testing early after myocardial infarction: Historic perspective and current use. *Prog Cardiovasc Dis 28*:463–476, 1986.
16. Hanson P: Clinical exercise testing. In *Sports Medicine.* Edited by R Strauss. Philadelphia: W.B. Saunders Co., 1984.

17. Haskell W, Brachfeld N, Bruce RA, Davis PO, Dennis CA, Fox SM, Hanson P and Leon AS: Task Force II: Determination of occupational working capacity in patients with ischemic heart disease. *JACC 14*:1025–1034, 1989.
18. Hollenberg M, Zolltick JM, Go M, Yaney SF, Daniels W, Davis RC and Bedynek JL: Comparison of a quantitative treadmill exercise score with standard electrocardiographic criteria in screening asymptomatic young men for coronary artery disease. *N Engl J Med 313*:600–606, 1985.
19. Klingfield P, Ameisen O and Okin PM: Heart rate adjustment of ST segment depression for improved detection of coronary artery disease. *Circulation 79*:245–255, 1989.
20. Ladenheim ML, Kotler TS, Pollock BH, Berman DS and Diamond GS: Incremental prognostic power of clinical history, exercise electrocardiography and myocardial perfusion scintigraphy in suspected coronary artery disease. *Am J Cardiol 59*:270–277, 1987.
21. Mark DB, Hlatky MA, Harrell FE, Lee KL, Califf RM and Pryor DB: Exercise treadmill score for predicting prognosis in coronary artery disease. *Ann Intern Med 106*:793–800, 1987.
22. Mark DB, Hlatkey MA, Lee KL, Harrell FE, Califf RM and Pryor DB: Localizing coronary obstructions with the treadmill test. *Ann Intern Med 106*:53–55, 1988.
23. Schauer JE and Hanson P: Usefulness of a branching treadmill protocol for evaluation of cardiac functional capacity. *Am J Cardiol 60*:1373–1377, 1987.
24. Weber KT and Janicki JS: Cardiopulmonary testing for the evaluation of chronic cardiac failure. *Am J Cardiol 55*:22A–31A, 1985.
25. Weiner DA, McCabe CH and Ryan TJ: Identification of patients with left main and three vessel coronary disease with clinical and exercise test variables. *Am J Cardiol 46*:21–27, 1980.
26. Weiner DA, Ryan TJ, McCabe CH, Kennedy JW, Schloss M, Tristani F, Chaitman BR and Fisher LD: Exercise stress testing: Correlations among history of angina, ST segment response and prevalence of coronary artery disease in the Coronary Artery Surgery Study (CASS). *N Engl J Med 301*:230–235, 1979.

BOOKS

27. Ellestad MH: *Stress Testing: Principles and Practice,* 3rd Ed. Baltimore: Williams & Wilkins, 1986.
28. Froelicher V: *Exercise and the Heart,* 2nd Ed. Chicago, IL: Year Book Publishers, Inc., 1987.
29. Wasserman K, Hanson JE, Sue DY and Whipp BJ: *Principles of Exercise Testing and Interpretation.* Philadelphia: Lea & Febiger, 1987.
30. Weber K and Janicki JS: *Cardiopulmonary Exercise Testing.* Philadelphia: W.B. Saunders Co., 1986.

CHAPTER 5

Principles of Exercise Prescription

"Exercise prescription" is the process whereby a person's recommended regimen of physical activity is designed in a systematic and individualized manner. An exercise prescription should designate the mode, intensity, duration, frequency, and progression of physical activity. These five components are applicable to the development of exercise programs for persons regardless of age, functional capacity, and presence or absence of disease states. The appropriate exercise prescription for any individual is best determined from an objective evaluation of physical fitness including observations of heart rate, ECG, arterial blood pressure, and functional capacity obtained during an exercise test. However, as was discussed in Chapter 1, in most persons an exercise test is not required before initiation of an exercise program. In all cases, the exercise prescription should be developed with careful consideration of individual health history, risk factor profile, behavioral characteristics, and personal goals and preferences.

This chapter presents the general principles that should be applied in developing exercise prescriptions to enhance the health related components of physical fitness (i.e., cardiorespiratory endurance, body composition, flexibility, and muscular strength and endurance). Subsequent chapters address the specific considerations that pertain to exercise prescription for cardiac patients and others with special exercise needs.

PURPOSES OF EXERCISE PRESCRIPTION

The specific purposes of an exercise prescription vary with the individual's interest, needs, background, and health status. In most cases the exercise prescription is designed to: (1) enhance physical fitness, (2) promote health by reducing risk for future development or recurrence of disease, and (3) ensure safety during participation in exercise. These common purposes for prescribing exercise do not carry equal or consistent weight in all exercise programs or with all persons. In some cases enhancement of physical fitness may be the primary goal; in other instances, reduction of risk for disease may be the central concern. Exercise prescriptions can and should reflect the specific outcomes that are sought by a particular person.

Traditional approaches to development of the exercise prescription have been based largely on the body of knowledge that links increased exercise participation to improved physical fitness. Research has led to identification and acceptance of general procedures for enhancement of maximal aerobic power ($\dot{V}O_{2max}$) and muscular strength. These procedures have been presented in previous editions of this publication and in Position Stands of the American College of Sports Medicine.[1,2] Much less is known about exercise prescription for the purpose of reducing specific disease risks. However, recent research indicates that the amount of exercise needed to significantly reduce disease risk may be considerably less than that needed to develop and maintain high levels of physical fitness.[3] This observation carries important implications for health professionals who prescribe exercise for their clients and patients. The key implication is that levels of physical activity below those corresponding to the amount needed to enhance fitness may be the most appropriate target for some persons. Certainly, the amount of exercise associated with significantly enhanced fitness is desirable in most individuals. However, public health surveys indicate that a small percentage of adults attain that amount. For the sedentary person adoption of a *moderately active* lifestyle may carry important health benefits and may be a much more attainable goal than achievement of high levels of activity and fitness.

THE ART OF EXERCISE PRESCRIPTION

The guidelines for exercise prescription presented in this book are based on a solid foundation of scientific information. However, the pertinent body of knowledge is not so extensive as to support its application in a highly rigid and precise fashion. As suggested by the title of this chapter, the procedures recommended below are *principles.* They are *not* theorems or laws. Accordingly, the techniques presented should be utilized with flexibility and with careful attention to the characteristics and goals of the individual.

The physiological and perceptual responses to acute exercise vary considerably across individuals. Likewise, in different persons the adaptations to exercise training vary in terms of magnitude and rate of development. Therefore, exercise program personnel should be prepared to modify exercise prescriptions in accordance with the responses and adaptations observed in individual participants. Also, it should be recognized that, in most persons, desirable outcomes can be attained with exercise programs that vary considerably in terms of mode, frequency, duration, and intensity. Accordingly, development and implementation of exercise prescriptions in a rigid, mathematic fashion may be inappropriate. The fundamental objective of exercise prescription is to aid participants in increasing their habitual physical activity. The most appropriate exercise prescription for a particular person is the one that is most helpful in achieving this behavior change. To be sure, the basic exercise prescription process is a scientific one. However, successful exercise programs apply the accepted scientific principles to individual persons in a flexible manner. Exercise program personnel should recognize that the process of exercise prescription is an art as well as a science.

CARDIORESPIRATORY FITNESS

Based on the existing evidence concerning exercise prescription for enhancement of health and cardiorespiratory fitness, the following recommendations for the quantity and quality of endurance exercise are made. These recommendations are similar but not identical to those found in the American College of Sports Medicine's Position Stand on the recommended quantity and quality of exercise for developing and maintaining cardiorespiratory and muscular fitness in healthy adults.[1] The two sets of recommendations are not identical because the Position Stand focuses primarily on fitness enhancement, whereas the recommendations summarized below are designed to encompass activity that may enhance health without having a major impact on fitness.

- Mode of activity: Any activity that uses large muscle groups, that can be maintained for a prolonged period, and is rhythmic and aerobic in nature, e.g., running-jogging, walking-hiking, swimming, skating, bicycling, rowing, cross-country skiing, rope skipping, or various endurance game activities.

- Intensity of exercise: Physical activity corresponding to 40 to 85% $\dot{V}O_{2max}$ or 55 to 90% of maximal heart rate. It should be noted that exercise of lower intensity may provide important health benefits and may result in increased fitness in some persons (e.g., those who were previously sedentary and low fit).
- Duration of exercise: 15 to 60 minutes of continuous or discontinuous aerobic activity.
- Frequency of exercise: 3 to 5 days per week.
- Rate of progression: In most cases, the conditioning effect allows individuals to increase the total work done per session. In continuous exercise this occurs by an increase in intensity, duration, or by some combination of the two. The most significant conditioning effects may be observed during the first 6 to 8 weeks of the exercise program. The exercise prescription may be adjusted as these conditioning effects occur with the adjustment depending on participant characteristics, new exercise test results and/or exercise performance during exercise sessions.

The components of an exercise prescription listed above are interdependent. For example, the recommended duration of exercise is, in part, a function of intensity and frequency. Similar conditioning effects can be expected with exercise programs that involve comparable total amounts of activity (i.e., caloric expenditure) quantified on a weekly basis. Within the recommended ranges, frequency, intensity, and duration of exercise can be adjusted so as to provide the desired weekly caloric expenditure.

The principles of prescribing exercise for cardiorespiratory fitness are similar for asymptomatic and symptomatic participants. Differences arise in the manner in which the principles are applied, i.e., higher intensity vs. lower intensity, longer duration vs. short duration, daily exercise vs. 3 times per week, and use of symptomatology in determining exercise limits. For asymptomatic, physically active young people, modifications in intensity and duration of exercise are a simple matter involving minimal risk. Individualization of the exercise prescription is more important with sedentary, older, pregnant, or symptomatic participants and those with known disease (see

Chapters 6 and 7). In prescribing exercise for such individuals risk status should be considered carefully. The risks of exercise are reviewed in Chapter 1.

CARDIORESPIRATORY ENDURANCE ACTIVITIES

A key purpose of most exercise prescriptions is to increase or maintain functional capacity. To accomplish this goal a portion of each exercise session is devoted to aerobic endurance activities.

Endurance activities may be classified on the basis of: (a) inter-individual variability in caloric expenditure (i.e., economy or oxygen cost), and (b) potential for maintenance of a constant rate of energy expenditure. Some activities (Group 1), like walking, jogging, or cycling can be readily maintained at a constant intensity and inter-individual variability in energy expenditure is relatively low. For other activities (Group 2), such as swimming or cross-country skiing, the rate of energy expenditure is highly related to skill, but for a given individual can provide a constant intensity. Still other activities (Group 3), such as dancing, basketball, and racquetball, etc. are, by nature, highly variable in intensity.

When precise control of exercise intensity is necessary, as in the early stages of a rehabilitation program, Group 1 and 2 activities are recommended. Individual fitness levels and personal preference determine whether Group 1 and 2 activities are performed in a continuous or discontinuous (interval conditioning) exercise format. These activities continue to be useful at all stages of a conditioning program because they require relatively high rates of energy expenditure. Group 3 activities can be extremely useful because of the enjoyment provided in a physically active setting and because they may direct the participant's attention away from anxieties, worries, and boredom. However, such activities should be applied cautiously with high risk, symptomatic and low fit participants. Competitive aspects of games should be minimized. Also, before engaging in these activities patients in rehabilitation programs should: (1) demonstrate stable responses to exercise, and (2) be capable of sustaining an exercise intensity of approximately 5 METs.

INTENSITY OF EXERCISE

The most difficult problem in designing exercise programs is the prescription of the appropriate exercise intensity. This requires individualization and adequate monitoring to ensure that the maximum prescribed intensity is not exceeded. The intensity of exercise may be expressed in either absolute (e.g., watts) or relative terms (percentage of functional capacity). Usually exercise intensity is prescribed as a percentage of individual functional capacity using heart rate, rating of perceived exertion (RPE), METs, or estimated energy expenditure ($\dot{V}O_2$) as the means for making adjustments to the desired relative intensity.

The percentage of functional capacity a given individual is able to sustain for a specified conditioning period is quite variable. Marathon runners are able to maintain 80% of their $\dot{V}O_{2max}$ for over 2 hours, but poorly conditioned individuals exercising at 80% are fatigued in a few minutes. This variance may be explained in part by differences in the relative intensity of exercise at which the onset of blood lactate accumulation (OBLA) occurs. These differences in the ability to sustain a given exercise intensity must be taken into consideration in developing the exercise prescription.

In general, exercise during conditioning sessions should be prescribed at an intensity within the range of 40 to 85% of functional capacity. Typically, the conditioning intensity for healthy adults is between 60 and 70% of functional capacity. Participants, including cardiac patients, who have a low functional capacity, may initiate their conditioning at 40 to 60% of their functional capacity. Duration can then be set empirically, based on individual responses. For example, the participant should feel rested and not fatigued within an hour following exercise.

PRINCIPLES OF INTENSITY PRESCRIPTION

Various techniques can be used to prescribe and monitor exercise intensity. Among these are heart rate, RPE, and the designation of physical activities that require known rates of energy expenditure, i.e., those in which the MET values are predictable. Regardless of the specific procedure used, the central purpose is to monitor and thereby control the intensity of exercise in the range determined to be appropriate for the individual participant that allows 15 to 60 minutes of activity to be completed. The purpose of this process of developing an intensity prescription is to use the heart rate, RPE, or MET value to *guide* the participant in performing exercise at the appropriate intensity consistent with increasing or maintaining functioning capacity.

As was noted above, exercise intensity should typically be prescribed in the range of 40 to 85% of functional capacity. However, the intensity prescription should also consider the current exercise habits of the individual, i.e., a low fit and currently sedentary individual would exercise at a lower average percent of functional capacity than someone who is currently active and has a higher functional capacity. In addition, medical conditions, e.g., orthopedic limitations or obesity, would also suggest a lower intensity, with the provision of weight supported work. It must be emphasized that while the training intensity might average 70% of functional capacity, the individual will typically exercise 10% above and below that value in an exercise session. It is therefore customary to provide a range or "window" of training intensities consistent with achieving or maintaining functional capacity.

EXERCISE PRESCRIPTION BY HEART RATE

In general, unless disturbed by environmental conditions, psychological stimuli or disease, a relatively linear relationship exists between heart rate and exercise intensity. Individual differences in the heart rate-exercise intensity relationship can be detected during an exercise test.

There are several acceptable methods for calculating an appropriate "target" heart rate range. The first is to plot the line that shows the relationship between the exercise heart rate and $\dot{V}O_2$, expressed in either METs or $\dot{V}O_2$ (Fig. 5–1). The "maximal" heart rate is usually the heart rate measured at the highest exercise intensity attained during a maximal exercise test. From this relationship, the range of heart rates associated with given percentages of functional capacity can be determined. A target heart rate range may be used for regulating intensity during conditioning.

The second method used to determine the target heart rate range for a participant takes a percent of the difference between the maximal and the resting heart rates (heart rate range or reserve). It has been determined that 60 to 80% of the heart rate range corresponds to approximately 60 to 80% of the functional capacity. A target heart rate range for an asymptomatic person who has a maximal heart rate of 180 beats·min^{-1} and a resting heart rate of 60 beats·min^{-1} follows:

Target Heart Rate Range

	Lower Limit	*Upper Limit*
Maximal heart rate	180	180
Resting heart rate	− 60	− 60
Heart rate reserve	120	120
Conditioning intensity (60–80% HR range)	× .60	× .80
	72	96
Resting heart rate	+ 60	+ 60
Target heart rate	132	156

The third method for determining the target heart rate range simply takes a fixed percent of the maximal heart rate. This procedure is based on the observation that 70 and 85% of maximal heart rate is equal to about 60 and 80% of functional capacity. For example, for the person with a maximal heart rate of 180 beats$\cdot$min^{-1}, the target heart rate range calculated by this method is 126 and 153 beats$\cdot$min^{-1} (70% and 85% of 180 beats$\cdot$min^{-1}). These values are quite similar to those given by the heart rate range method described above. No matter what method is used, the target heart rate range is only a *guideline* to follow in prescribing exercise. The exercise leader must use judgment about how a given individual is responding to the exercise, and alter the intensity to provide for the participant's comfort and safety while trying to achieve a training effect and the expenditure of a large number of calories.

The target heart rates calculated by the procedures outlined above are applicable to most activities in which a steady-state is attained and under most environmental conditions. In discontinuous exercise, the alternating higher and lower energy demands may be accompanied by heart rates 10% higher and 10% lower than the average target heart rate. However, the exercise intervals should be of such duration that the heart rate, over time, averages out to a value near the mid-point of the prescribed range.

Heart rate can be determined from measurements made during ECG monitoring, radiotelemetry, or palpation. The latter two methods are more adaptable to nonlaboratory situations, with the palpation technique better suited to large groups.

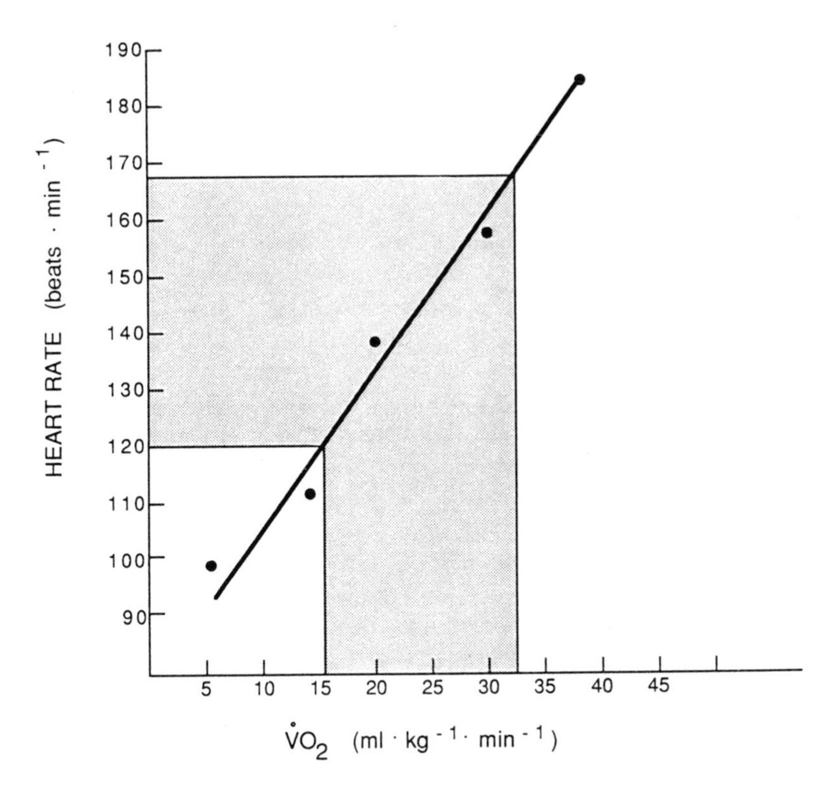

FIGURE 5–1. A line of best fit has been drawn through the data points on this plot of heart rate and oxygen consumption data observed during a hypothetical maximal exercise test in which $\dot{V}O_{2max}$ was observed to be 38 ml·kg^{-1}·min^{-1} and maximal heart rate was 184 beats·min^{-1}. A target heart rate range was determined by finding the heart rates that correspond to 40% and 85% of $\dot{V}O_{2max}$. For this individual, 40% of $\dot{V}O_{2max}$ was approximately 15 ml·kg^{-1}·min^{-1} and 85% of $\dot{V}O_{2max}$ was approximately 32 ml·kg^{-1}·min^{-1}. The corresponding heart rates are approximately 120 and 168 beats·min^{-1}. The target heart rate range for this individual is 120 to 168 beats·min^{-1}.

Counting the pulse for 10 (or 15) seconds immediately after a bout of exercise and multiplying by 6 (or 4) gives a good estimate of exercise heart rate.

EXERCISE PRESCRIPTION BY RPE

The commonly employed RPE scales are shown in Chapter 4. One is a 15-point numerical scale ranging from 6 to 20 with a verbal description provided at every odd number. The alternative is similar but uses a scale ranging from 1 to 10. The RPE response to graded exercise correlates highly with cardiorespiratory and metabolic variables such as $\dot{V}O_2$, heart rate, and ventilation. RPE is a valid and reliable indicator of the level of physical exertion during steady-state exercise and, therefore, can be used to establish an exercise intensity for endurance training.

Using the 15-point scale, a perceived exertion rating of 12 to 13 corresponds to approximately 60% of the heart rate range. A rating of 16 corresponds to approximately 85% of heart rate range. Consequently, most participants should exercise within the RPE range of 12 and 16 ("somewhat hard" to "hard"). Corresponding ratings using the 10-point RPE scale would be between 4 and 6. It should be noted that a small percentage of participants (~10%) tend to select abnormal or unrealistic RPE scores and, in these persons, the RPE method for exercise prescription may be inappropriate.

The individual participant's RPE response to graded exercise may be employed in specifying the RPE level for conditioning. Also, RPE can be used in conjunction with heart rate prescription methods. At the onset of a training program the participant can be instructed to exercise at a specified heart rate and to self-monitor the RPE at that intensity. After the participant has developed a knowledge of the heart rate-RPE relationship, heart rate can be monitored less frequently and RPE can be employed as the primary method for regulating intensity. In addition, changes in RPE can be used as a guideline in modifying the exercise prescription.

EXERCISE PRESCRIPTION BY METs

The mode of exercise may be selected by determining the desired range of percentages of the individual's functional capacity and then identifying activities that are known to require energy expenditure at a rate that falls within that range. Generally, 40 to 85% of functional capacity (maximal METs) is an appropriate range of conditioning intensities, although higher intensity ranges can be employed by persons with higher fitness levels.

Table 5–1 provides means and ranges for MET requirements of many of the common leisure activities. Appendix D also contains information on energy costs of selected activities.

Regardless of the prescriptive technique employed, the average exercise intensity during a given conditioning session may be obtained by alternating periods of exercise at higher and lower intensities. If, for example, an exercise intensity of 6 to 8 METs (or comparable heart rate or RPE) is prescribed, equal time intervals at 5 and 9 METs will result in an average rate of energy expenditure that falls in the desired range. When initiating an exercise program exercise intensity should be maintained near the lower end of the target range until the participant has become accustomed to exercise and the exercise leader is familiar with the participant's response.

For physical activities such as walking, jogging, running, cycle ergometer exercise, and stepping or stair climbing, the exercise intensity in METs is directly related to speed of movement or measurable resistance (see Appendix D). Even in these activities, the maintenance of the prescribed safe conditioning intensity can be complicated by changes in the environment. Critical environmental factors include: wind, hills, sand, snow, obstacles such as ditches, fences or underbrush, heat or cold, humidity, altitude, pollution, bulky clothing or clothing that obstructs movement, and the weight and size of equipment such as back packs, skis, suitcases, or grocery bags. Difficulties in maintaining a prescribed exercise intensity in a changing environment can usually be overcome by using heart rate or RPE as the indicator of exercise intensity. Prescription and maintenance of desired exercise intensities are more difficult in complex dual sports such as tennis, handball, or squash, and team sports such as volleyball, softball, soccer, or basketball. With such activities heart rate is a less reliable indicator of the rate of energy expenditure than in the case with steady-state activities like walking or cycling.

The exercise leader may use the MET prescription, heart rate prescription, RPE prescription or all in setting appropriate exercise intensities for various activities. As one adapts to conditioning, heart rate and RPE for a given MET level generally decrease; therefore, participants should increase their MET level progressively to correspond to their target heart rate or RPE. Periodic re-evaluation aids in measuring progress and updating the exercise prescription.

It is important to remember that intensity should be prescribed within a range regardless of the methods used. For example, if the percentage of heart rate range method is used, and a target range of 132 to 156 is calculated, one should expect a participant's exercise heart rate to fluctuate within that range.

Table 5–1. Leisure Activities in METs: Sports, Exercise Classes, Games, Dancing.

	Mean	*Range*
Archery	3.9	3–4
Back Packing	—	5–11
Badminton	5.8	4–9+
Basketball		
Gameplay	8.3	7–12+
Non-game	—	3–9
Billiards	2.5	—
Bowling	—	2–4
Boxing		
In-ring	13.3	—
Sparring	8.3	—
Canoeing, Rowing and Kayaking	—	3–8
Conditioning Exercise	—	3–8+
Climbing Hills	7.2	5–10+
Cricket	5.2	4.6–7.4
Croquet	3.5	—
Cycling		
Pleasure or to work	—	3–8+
10 mph	7.0	—
Dancing (Social, Square, Tap)	—	3.7–7.4
Dancing (Aerobic)	—	6–9
Fencing	—	6–10+
Field Hockey	8.0	—
Fishing		
from bank	3.7	2–4
wading in stream	—	5–6
Football (Touch)	7.9	6–10
Golf		
Power cart	—	2–3
Walking (carrying bag or pulling cart)	5.1	4–7
Handball	—	8–12+
Hiking (Cross-country)	—	3–7
Horseback Riding		
Galloping	8.2	—
Trotting	6.6	—
Walking	2.4	—
Horseshoe Pitching	—	2–3
Hunting (Bow or Gun)		
Small game (walking, carrying light load)	—	3–7
Big game (dragging carcass, walking)	—	3–14
Judo	13.5	—
Mountain Climbing	—	5–10+
Music Playing	—	2–3
Paddleball, Racquetball	9	8–12
Rope Jumping	11	—
60–80 skips/min	9	—
120–140 skips/min	—	11–12

Table 5–1. Leisure Activities in METs: Sports, Exercise Classes, Games, Dancing *(Continued).*

	Mean	*Range*
Running		
12 min per mile	8.7	—
11 min per mile	9.4	—
10 min per mile	10.2	—
9 min per mile	11.2	—
8 min per mile	12.5	—
7 min per mile	14.1	—
6 min per mile	16.3	—
Sailing	—	2–5
Scubadiving	—	5–10
Shuffleboard	—	2–3
Skating, Ice and Roller	—	5–8
Skiing, Snow		
Downhill	—	5–8
Crosscountry	—	6–12+
Skiing, Water	—	5–7
Sledding, Tobogganing	—	4–8
Snowshoeing	9.9	7–14
Squash	—	8–12+
Soccer	—	5–12+
Stairclimbing	—	4–8
Swimming	—	4–8+
Table Tennis	4.1	3–5
Tennis	6.5	4–9+
Volleyball	—	3–6

Also, it should be anticipated that some individuals may not be able to comfortably tolerate the prescribed intensity, whereas others may find it much too easy. In such cases adjustments are appropriate and indeed necessary. Adjusting the individual's exercise intensity within a reasonable range is an important part of the art of exercise prescription.

Finally, it should be emphasized that the individual's signs and symptoms of CAD or other disease may be overriding factors in prescribing the intensity of exercise. As will be discussed in Chapters 6 and 7, certain manifestations of chronic disease (e.g., angina pectoris, intermittent claudication, chronic obstructive pulmonary disease) may require that exercise intensity be maintained at levels below those calculated using the standard procedures described above.

DURATION OF THE EXERCISE SESSION

The conditioning period, exclusive of warm-up and cool-down, may vary in length from 15 to 60 minutes. Most typically the conditioning phase is 20 to 30 minutes. This length of time is required to improve or maintain functional capacity. The appropriate duration of the conditioning period is inversely related to the intensity of the exercise expressed as a percentage of the functional capacity. The conditioning response resulting from an exercise program is a result of the product of the intensity and the duration of exercise (total energy expenditure). Significant cardiovascular improvements have been obtained with exercise sessions of 5 to 10 minutes' duration with an intensity of more than 90% of functional capacity. However, high intensity-short duration sessions are not desirable for most participants and better results are obtained with lower intensities and longer durations. Such programs are preferred because they may carry lower risk of orthopedic injury and involve a relatively high total caloric expenditure.

For sedentary, asymptomatic, and symptomatic participants exercise sessions of moderate duration (20 to 30 minutes) and moderate intensity (40 to 60% of functional capacity) are advisable during the first weeks of conditioning. Multiple short bouts (~10 minutes) of exercise distributed throughout the day may be optimal for some participants. Changes in the exercise prescription must be made as the individual's functional capacity increases and as physiological adaptation to exercise occurs. Modification of the duration-intensity level should be individualized on the basis of the subject's functional capacity, health status, goals (e.g., weight loss) and response to specific exercise activities. If a normal conditioning response is obtained with no complications, the duration may be increased gradually from 20 to 45 minutes during the initial stage of a conditioning program.

FREQUENCY OF EXERCISE SESSIONS

The frequency of exercise depends in part on the duration and intensity of the exercise session. The recommended frequency varies from several daily sessions, to 3 to 5 periods per week according to the needs, interests and functional capacity of the participants. For some individuals with functional capacities less than 3 METs, sessions of 5 minutes' duration several times daily may be desirable. For persons with capacities between 3 and 5 METs, 1 to 2 daily sessions may be advisable. Typically participants with capacities of more than 5 METs should exercise at least 3 times per week on alternate days.

However, some persons in this category may benefit most from a program that involves moderate doses of exercise on a daily basis.

In the first few weeks of a program that uses weight-bearing exercise, it is desirable to alternate a day of exercise with a day of rest. Another desirable approach involves exercise on 5 or more days per week, but with alternation between weight-bearing and nonweight-bearing activities.

RATE OF PROGRESSION

The recommended rate of progression in the exercise conditioning program depends on the individual's functional capacity, health status, age, preferences and needs or goals. The endurance or aerobic phase of the exercise prescription has three stages of progression: initial, improvement, and maintenance.

INITIAL CONDITIONING STAGE

The initial stage should include light calisthenics and low level aerobic activities with which the participant experiences a minimum of muscle soreness and avoids debilitating injuries or discomfort. Discomfort is often associated with starting an exercise program without adequate time for physiological adaptation. Program compliance may be reduced if a program is initiated too abruptly. It may help to start with an exercise intensity approximately 1 MET lower than that estimated at 40 to 85% of the functional capacity. For example, a calculated exercise intensity range of 7 to 9 METs might be set initially at a more conservative 6 METs. If the participant selects a jogging program, information in Appendix D indicates that a 4-mph pace would be appropriate. A cycle ergometer program might also be suggested for this 70-kg participant at 100 Watts. The validity of these estimates of intensity should always be checked by having the participants, unless symptom limited, exercise at these intensities for a minimum of 3 minutes and then checking the pulse. Exercise intensities may require adjustment; lower intensity if the participant is above the target heart rate range, and higher intensity if the participant is below the target range. With conditioning, heart rate decreases for a given exercise intensity. Therefore, the heart rate (used in combination with signs and symptoms) is one of the best indicators that the participant's exercise prescription should be adjusted to the next level. A combination of objective and subjective factors must be considered when progressing individuals in their exercise routines.

Initially, the duration of the aerobic conditioning phase of the exercise prescription should be at least 10 to 15 minutes and should be gradually increased. Beginning frequency depends on the participant's functional capacity (Table 5–2). The initial conditioning stage usually lasts from 4 to 6 weeks, but this is dependent upon the rate of adaptation of the participant to the program. For example, a person who has a low fitness level or who is limited by CAD may spend as many as 6 to 10 weeks in the initial phase, while the participant with a higher fitness level may not need to participate more than a few weeks in the initial phase or may be exempted from this stage if already engaged in an exercise program.

Health status must also be considered in the rate of progression. For example, patients with symptoms of exertional angina during the initial stage may have to exercise for a period of time at 40 to 50% of functional capacity. Persons with intermittent claudication may only be able to tolerate 1 to 2 minutes of exercise alternated with rest periods. Following a debilitating illness or major surgical procedure functional capacities are often as low as 2 or 3 METs. Initially, exercise duration may be less than 5 minutes due to angina, local muscle fatigue, or breathlessness. The necessity for individual modifications cannot be overemphasized, although no attempt can be made to provide a list of all the possible modifications for all participants. More detail on this issue is provided in Chapters 6 and 7.

At the onset of an exercise program individual goals should be established. These goals should be developed by the participant with the guidance of the fitness instructor or exercise specialist. A key is to establish goals that are realistic. Also, a

Table 5–2. Cardiorespiratory Fitness Levels.*

Fitness Level	$\dot{V}O_2$ $ml \cdot kg^{-1} \cdot min^{-1}$	*METs*
Poor	3.5–13.9	1.0–3.9
Low	14.0–24.9	4.0–6.9
Average	25.0–38.9	7.0–10.9
Good	39.0–48.9	11.0–13.9
High	49.0–56.0	14.0–16.0

*For 40-year-old males. Adjustments are appropriate to apply these standards to others.

system of rewards, tangible or intangible, should be established at this time.

IMPROVEMENT CONDITIONING STAGE

The improvement stage of the aerobic phase of the exercise conditioning program differs from the initial stage in that the participant is progressed at a more rapid rate. This stage typically lasts for 4 to 5 months. During this stage intensity is increased to the target level within the 40 to 85% $\dot{V}O_{2max}$ range. Duration is increased consistently every 2 to 3 weeks. The frequency and magnitude of the increments are dictated by the rate at which the participant adapts to the conditioning program. Cardiac patients and less fit individuals should be permitted more time for adaptation at each stage of conditioning. It is recommended that symptom limited participants initially use discontinuous aerobic exercise and progress toward continuous aerobic exercise. The duration of exercise for these participants should be increased to 20 to 30 minutes before increasing the intensity (Table 5–3).

Age must also be taken into consideration when progressions are recommended. Experience suggests that adaptation to conditioning may take longer in older individuals.

MAINTENANCE CONDITIONING STAGE

The maintenance stage of the exercise prescription usually begins after the first 6 months of training. During the maintenance stage the participant usually reaches a satisfactory level of cardiorespiratory fitness and may no longer be interested in increasing the conditioning load. While further improvement may be minimal, continuing the same workout schedule enables one to maintain fitness.

At this point, the objectives of conditioning should be reviewed and realistic goals set. To maintain fitness, a specific exercise program should be designed that will be similar in energy cost to the conditioning program and also satisfy the needs of the participant over a long time span. More enjoyable or variable activities may be substituted for those used in the improvement stage. This may help avoid participant dropout which often results when activities become boring due to repetition.

Table 5–3. Example: Progression of the Symptomatic Participant Using a Discontinuous Aerobic Conditioning Phase.*

Endurance/ Aerobic Phase	*Weeks*	*Total Minutes at % FC†*	*% FC*	*Minutes at Exercise Intensity (60–80% FC)*	*Minutes at Rest Phase Lower than Exercise Intensity*	*Repetitions*
Initial Stage	1	12	60	2	1	6
	2	14	60	2	1	7
	3	16	60	2	1	8
	4	18	60–70	2	1	9
	5	20	60–70	2	1	10
Improvement Stage	6–9	21	70–80	3	1	7
	10–13	24	70–80	3	1	8
	14–16	24	70–80	4	1	6
	17–19	28	70–80	4	1	7
	20–23	30	70–80	5	1	6
	24–27	30	70–80	Continuous		
Maintenance Stage	28+	45–60	70–80	Continuous		

*Clinical status must be considered before advancing to the next level
†FC—Functional Capacity

FLEXIBILITY

Normal musculoskeletal function requires that an adequate range of motion be maintained in all joints. Of particular concern is maintenance of flexibility in the lower back/posterior thigh region. Lack of flexibility in this region may be associated with increased risk for development of chronic lower back pain. Therefore, preventive and rehabilitative exercise programs should include activities that promote maintenance of good flexibility, particularly in the lower back. Lack of flexibility is particularly prevalent in the elderly among whom this condition often contributes to reduced ability to perform the activities of daily living. Accordingly, exercise programs for the elderly should emphasize proper stretching exercise, particularly for the upper and lower trunk, neck and hip regions.

Stretching exercises can aid in improving and maintaining range of motion in a joint or series of joints. Flexibility exercises should be performed slowly with a gradual progression to greater ranges of motion. A slow dynamic movement should be followed with a static stretch that is sustained for 10 to 30 seconds. Three to 5 repetitions of each exercise are recommended. The degree of stretch should not be so extreme as to cause significant pain. Stretching exercises should be performed at least 3 times per week and can be effectively included in the warm-up and/or cool-down periods that precede and follow the aerobic conditioning phase of an exercise session. It is recommended that an active warm-up precede vigorous stretching exercises. Therefore, if stretching exercises are performed prior to the aerobic exercise component of an activity session, they should be used with particular caution.

Stretching exercises for the posterior thigh and lower leg muscles may be helpful in preventing certain musculoskeletal injuries in the lower extremities. Moderate static stretching exercise also may be useful in relieving neuromuscular tension.

Some commonly employed stretching exercises may place participants at risk for musculoskeletal injuries. This concern is particularly important among participants who are relatively inflexible and/or who are novice exercisers. While research evidence concerning the risks of specific exercises is lacking, those activities that require substantial flexibility and/or skill are not recommended for older, less flexible and less experienced participants.

MUSCULAR STRENGTH AND ENDURANCE

Muscular strength and endurance have little direct relationship to cardiorespiratory fitness or functional capacity. However, many leisure and occupational tasks require arm exercise, e.g., moving, lifting, or holding a heavy object. The physiological stress induced by lifting or holding a given weight is proportional to the percentage of maximal strength involved. The maintenance or enhancement of muscle strength and muscle endurance enables the individual to perform such tasks with less physiological stress. Maintenance of adequate strength becomes an increasingly important issue with advancing age which is associated with a loss of lean weight.

Muscular strength is acquired either by dynamic high-tension low-repetition exercises or through static contractions. Both dynamic lifting procedures and static contractions result in an increased systemic arterial blood pressure. An increased blood pressure increases the work of the heart and its requirements for oxygen. Such lifts may cause a reduction in venous return and result in decreased blood flow to the heart and brain if performed with the Valsalva maneuver. Therefore, maximal tension exercises should be discouraged for symptomatic or high risk individuals. Instead, dynamic low-weight exercises should be incorporated into the program for improvement of both muscle strength and endurance. If such activities are used, participants should be trained to perform the movements while breathing freely and rhythmically without breath-holding. Exhalation on effort should be encouraged. In addition, special attention should be directed toward sufficient warm-up and cool-down, correct body positioning for lifting, and rhythmic performance of the movements.

Strengthening exercises should be performed 2 to 3 times per week. Resistance may be applied to isotonically contracting muscles using free-weights, supported weight machines, or calisthenic exercises. Specially designed instruments can be employed to apply accommodating resistance during performance of dynamic muscle contractions or to allow performance of isokinetic muscle contractions (i.e., those performed at constant angular velocity). Optimal rates of strength gain occur when the established resistance allows no more than 5 to 7 repetitions of a movement and when three sets of the exercise are performed in a training session. However, significant strength gains can occur with exercises that apply lower levels of resistance (e.g., calisthenic exercises). It should be emphasized that high resistances are to be avoided with high risk, symptomatic and CAD patients.

PROGRAMS FOR REDUCING BODY FATNESS

An excessive percentage of body fat (% fat) may be associated with increased risk for development of hypertension, diabetes, CAD and other chronic diseases. Recent evidence indicates that "central obesity" (fat deposited primarily in the trunk-abdominal region) is particularly problematic. In addition, obesity often carries a negative social stigma and is associated with a reduced physical working capacity. Many participants in preventive and rehabilitative exercise programs are excessively fat. Since reduction of body fatness is a need and/or a goal of many exercise program participants, exercise prescriptions should be designed to aid in accomplishing this end. This section presents the principles that should be employed in modifying body composition.

CALORIC BALANCE

Body composition is determined by a complex set of genetic and behavioral factors. Though the contributing variables are many, the fundamental determinant of body weight and body composition is caloric balance. Caloric balance refers to the difference between caloric intake (energy equivalent of food ingested) and caloric expenditure (energy equivalent of biological work performed). It should be noted that factors such as meal distribution, food sources of calories, absolute caloric intake and basal metabolic rate may affect total caloric expenditure.

The First Law of Thermodynamics indicates that energy is neither created nor destroyed but may change form. Therefore, body weight is lost when caloric expenditure exceeds caloric intake (negative balance) and weight is gained when the opposite situation exists. It is known that one pound of fat is equivalent to approximately 3500 kcal of energy (1 kg $\approx$ 7700 kcal). Though it is predictable that shifts in caloric balance will be accompanied by changes in body weight, the nature of a weight change varies markedly with the specific behaviors that lead to a caloric imbalance. For example, fasting and extreme caloric restriction diets cause substantial losses of water and lean tissue. In contrast, an exercise-induced negative caloric balance results in weight losses that consist primarily of adipose tissue. High resistance exercise programs (e.g., weight lifting) may lead to a gain in lean weight, while aerobic training usually results only in a maintenance of lean weight. Both types of programs can contribute to a loss of fat, although aerobic activity is more efficient because it involves a sustained, high rate of energy expenditure.

RECOMMENDED WEIGHT LOSS PROGRAMS

Substantial evidence indicates that, for most persons, the optimal approach to weight loss combines a mild caloric restriction with regular endurance exercise. A desirable weight loss program is one that meets the following criteria:

1. Provides intake not lower than 1200 $kcal \cdot d^{-1}$ for normal adults so as to provide a proper blend of foods to meet nutritional requirements. (Note: this requirement may change for children, older individuals, athletes, etc.).
2. Includes foods acceptable to the dieter in terms of sociocultural background, usual habits, taste, costs and ease in acquisition and preparation.
3. Provides a negative caloric balance (not to exceed 500 to 1000 $kcal \cdot d^{-1}$) resulting in gradual weight loss without metabolic derangements, such as ketosis. Maximal weight loss should be 1 $kg \cdot wk^{-1}$.
4. Includes the use of behavior modification techniques to identify and eliminate diet habits that contribute to improper nutrition.
5. Includes an exercise program that provides a daily caloric expenditure of 300 or more kcal. For many participants this may be best accomplished with exercise of low intensity but long duration, such as walking.
6. Provides that the new eating and physical activity habits can be continued for life in order to maintain the achieved lower body weight (see Chapter 8).

Weight loss programs that manifest the aforementioned characteristics have been shown to minimize nutritional deficiencies and losses of fat-free tissue that result from severe restrictions of caloric intake.

In designing the exercise component of a weight loss regimen, the principles presented earlier in this chapter should be employed. In weight loss programs the major goal of the exercise prescription is to increase caloric expenditure. Therefore, when exercise is prescribed for the primary purpose of promoting weight loss, the balance between intensity and duration of exercise should be manipulated so as to yield a high total caloric expenditure (300 to 500 kcal per session and 1000 to 2000 kcal per week for adults). Sustained aerobic activities are preferred because they cause the greatest total energy expenditure. Obese individuals are at an increased relative risk for orthopedic injury. This may require that the intensity of exercise be maintained at or below the 60% of functional capacity or maximal heart rate recommended for improvement of cardiorespiratory endurance. Nonweight-bearing activities (and/or rotation of exercise modes) may be necessary and modifications in frequency and duration may also be required.

THE EXERCISE SESSION

Each exercise session includes a warm-up of 5 to 10 minutes' duration; endurance (aerobic) activity lasting 15 to 60 minutes; and a cool-down of 5 to 10 minutes. Participants should be instructed to report any new illnesses or changes in symptoms at the beginning of the session. The warm-up period is designed to gradually increase the metabolic rate from the resting level of 1 MET to the MET level required for conditioning. The warm-up period usually lasts 5 to 10 minutes and may include walking or slow jogging, light stretching exercises, and calisthenics or other types of muscle conditioning exercises. The duration and intensity of each of these activities depends on environmental conditions, functional capacity, symptomatology, and exercise preferences of the participant. For participants who require or prefer greater amounts of muscle strength or endurance, additional calisthenics and exercises utilizing weights may be included. The endurance or aerobic phase of conditioning can be designed to be continuous or discontinuous. It includes aerobic-type activities involving large muscle groups to produce heart rates of prescribed intensity. Also, this phase of the exercise session may appropriately include a period of participation in recreational games. The cool-down period includes exercises of diminishing intensities, e.g., slower walking or jogging, stretching and in some cases, relaxation activities.

ENVIRONMENTAL FACTORS

The physiological responses to exercise may be profoundly affected by environmental factors such as extreme heat or cold, high altitude, terrain and air pollution. As the exercise environment varies, the exercise prescription should be modified so that physiological responses remain at the desired levels and the participant's health and safety are maintained. The exercise heart rate and RPE are useful methods of adjusting intensity for varying environmental conditions.

Environmental heat stress is a function of temperature, relative humidity, and radiant heating. Increased heat stress characteristically involves a greater sweat rate and cardiorespiratory response to a standard submaximal exercise load. Therefore, maintenance of a constant cardiorespiratory response necessitates a decrease in absolute exercise intensity. In extremely warm conditions duration of exercise should be restricted and care should be taken to adequately replace fluids during and after the exercise session. In extremely cold conditions the exerciser should provide protection against hypothermia and frost bite. Clothing should be worn that adequately protects the head and extremities. Whenever possible, symptomatic and high risk exercisers should exercise in moderate temperatures.

At high altitudes the partial pressure of oxygen in atmospheric air is reduced. This can impair systemic oxygen transport and cause an increased cardiorespiratory response to a standard submaximal exercise intensity. Therefore, upon ascent to higher altitudes (>1500 meters) the exercise prescription should be modified by decreasing the absolute exercise intensity and keeping heart rate and RPE constant.

High levels of air pollution may necessitate a restriction of the intensity and/or duration of exercise. This is of particular importance for patients with chronic pulmonary disease.

SPECIAL PRECAUTIONS

Since a primary purpose of most exercise prescriptions is to enhance participant health, it is important that exercise programs not cause or exacerbate health problems. Clearly participation in an exercise program carries some risk of incurring orthopedic injury. Unfortunately, the precise incidence of orthopedic injury and associated risk factors are not well understood for most forms of exercise. However, available research evidence and experience indicate that higher incidences of injury are associated with weight-bearing activities like jogging and running. Factors such as high exposure to exercise (e.g., high running mileage), personal history of injury, biomechanical deficiencies, and abrupt increases in exercise participation are associated with incidence of injury. Exercise program personnel should attempt to minimize participant risk of orthopedic injury by designing exercise prescriptions that provide moderate, gradually incremented doses of activity particularly in participants who are initiating exercise programs, who are obese and/or who have a history of injury with exercise. Non-weight bearing activities should be used preferentially with persons who are overweight and who have a history of lower extremity injury. Also, careful selection of footwear may be helpful.

The impact of regular exercise on risk of infectious illness is not well understood. Some evidence indicates that moderate exercise training may improve immune function, whereas extremely heavy exercise training may impair immune status. Also, relatively little is known about progression of existing infectious diseases such as upper respiratory illnesses. However, there are some reports of myocarditis developing in persons who continue to exercise heavily while suffering from such illnesses. Accordingly, it is recommended that vigorous exercise be avoided by persons who are experiencing infectious illnesses that are severe enough to be accompanied by fever or myalgia.

PROGRAM SUPERVISION

Health screening, medical evaluation, and exercise testing permit the classification of participants according to their capacity for participation in an unsupervised or supervised exercise program.

UNSUPERVISED EXERCISE PROGRAMS

Apparently healthy participants can usually exercise safely in an unsupervised conditioning program. Participants should be provided with individualized exercise prescriptions and should be made aware of the physiological effects of temperature, humidity, and altitude. Also, participants in unsupervised programs should be oriented to the signs of overexertion and should be instructed to seek professional consultation if symptoms of chronic disease manifest.

SUPERVISED EXERCISE PROGRAMS

A supervised exercise program is one that provides trained professional on-site leadership (e.g., health fitness instructor or preventive/rehabilitative exercise specialist). Such programs are particularly recommended for symptomatic and cardiorespiratory disease patients who are considered by their physicians to be clinically stable and who have been cleared by their physician for participation in the program. Also, these programs are useful for those who need instruction in proper exercise techniques and, in some participants, may enhance compliance with an exercise program. Although a signed informed consent is not mandatory, it may be useful in communicating the attendant risks and benefits of exercise.

MEDICALLY SUPERVISED EXERCISE PROGRAMS

A medically supervised exercise program is supervised directly by a physician or by trained professionals who are authorized and qualified to deliver emergency care and advanced cardiac life support. Such programs are most appropriate for: (1) cardiorespiratory patients who are initiating an exercise program, (2) patients who manifest unstable clinical profiles, and (3) higher risk, symptomatic, or chronic disease patients whose personal physician feels that medical supervision is required to ensure participant safety. Informed consent must be obtained in medically supervised programs (Appendix C).

REFERENCES

1. American College of Sports Medicine: Position stand on the recommended quantity and quality of exercise for developing and maintaining cardiorespiratory and muscular fitness in healthy adults. *Med Sci Sports Exerc 22*:265–274, 1990.
2. American College of Sports Medicine: Position statement on proper and improper weight loss programs. *Med Sci Sports Exerc 15*:ix–xiii, 1983.
3. Blair SN, Kohl HW, Paffenbarger RS, Clark DG, Cooper KH and Gibbons LW: Physical fitness and all-cause mortality: A prospective study of healthy men and women. *JAMA 262*:2395–2401, 1989.
4. Brownell KD: Weight management and body composition. In *Resource Manual for Guidelines for Exercise Testing and Prescription.* Edited by American College of Sports Medicine. Philadelphia: Lea & Febiger, 1988.
5. Committee on Exercise: *Exercise Testing and Training of Apparently Healthy Individuals: A Handbook for Physicians.* New York: American Heart Association, 1972.
6. Giese M: Organization of an exercise session. In *Resource Manual for Guidelines for Exercise Testing and Prescription.* Edited by American College of Sports Medicine. Philadelphia: Lea & Febiger, 1988.

7. Golding LA, Myers CR and Sinning WE (eds.): *Y's Way to Physical Fitness,* 3rd edition. Champaign, IL: Human Kinetics Publishers, 1989.
8. Howley ET and Franks BD: *Health/Fitness Instructor's Handbook.* Champaign, IL: Human Kinetics Publishers, 1986.
9. Leon AS, Connett J, Jacobs DR and Rauramaa R: Leisure-time physical activity levels and risk of coronary heart disease and death: The Multiple Risk Factor Intervention Trial. *JAMA 258*:2388–2395, 1987.
10. Melleby A: *The Y's Way to a Healthy Back.* Piscataway, NJ: New Century Publishers, 1982.
11. Moffatt RJ: Strength and flexibility considerations for exercise prescription. In *Resource Manual for Guidelines for Exercise Testing and Prescription.* Edited by American College of Sports Medicine. Philadelphia: Lea & Febiger, 1988.
12. Noble BJ: Clinical applications of perceived exertion. *Med Sci Sports Exerc 14*:406–411, 1982.
13. Paffenbarger RS, Jr, Hyde RT, Wing AL and Hsieh C-C: Physical activity, all-cause mortality, and longevity of college alumni. *N Engl J Med 314*:605–613, 1986.
14. Painter P and Haskell WL: Decision making in programming exercise. In *Resource Manual for Guidelines for Exercise Testing and Prescription.* Edited by American College of Sports Medicine. Philadelphia: Lea & Febiger, 1988.
15. Pollock ML, Wilmore JH and Fox SM: *Exercise in Health and Disease.* Philadelphia: WB Saunders Co., 1984.
16. Porter GH: Case study evaluation for exercise prescription. In *Resource Manual for Guidelines for Exercise Testing and Prescription.* Edited by American College of Sports Medicine. Philadelphia: Lea & Febiger, 1988.
17. Vogel JA, Jones BH and Rock PB: Environmental considerations in exercise testing and training. In *Resource Manual for Guidelines for Exercise Testing and Prescription.* Edited by American College of Sports Medicine. Philadelphia: Lea & Febiger, 1988.

Chapter 6

Exercise Prescription for Cardiac Patients

Cardiac rehabilitation is a multiphasic program of medical care that is designed to restore the coronary artery diseased (CAD) patient to a full and productive life. Programs are concerned with the physiological, psychological, social, vocational, and recreational aspects of human function. The following interventions should be included in many cardiac rehabilitation programs: exercise therapy, psychological counseling, vocational counseling, and behavioral intervention regimens to facilitate dietary change, smoking cessation, and stress management. All programs provide medical surveillance of the rehabilitation patient. In recent years, exercise training has become a widely accepted therapeutic modality for CAD patients and has become a central focus in many cardiac rehabilitation programs. The general principles of exercise prescription as discussed in Chapter 5 apply to CAD patients as well as to healthy persons. However, the physiological limitations imposed by CAD require that particular care be taken to individualize the exercise prescription in accordance with the patient's health history and clinical status. This chapter is designed to present the guidelines that should be employed in prescribing exercise for cardiac patients of various classes. The material in this chapter has been organized by dividing the rehabilitative process into three major phases: Inpatient (Phase I), Outpatient (Phase II), and Community programs (Phase III). However, it is recognized that cardiac rehabilitation programs can appropriately be divided into four or more phases.

TYPES OF CARDIAC PATIENTS

Cardiac patients vary in severity of atherosclerotic disease, impairment of ventricular function, functional capacity, occurrence of signs and symptoms, and clinical manifestations of disease (e.g., ischemia, abnormal blood pressure response). A rehabilitation program may include patients who have had coronary artery bypass surgery, myocardial infarction (MI), pacemaker implantation, valve replacement, cardiac transplant, or percutaneous transluminal coronary angioplasty (PTCA); or who have other evidence of cardiovascular disease such as angina pectoris or a positive exercise test, or evidence of disease from radionuclide study or coronary angiography. Emphasis should be placed on developing goals for recovery of the patient that are realistic and consistent with limitations imposed by the disease process. All patients need some level of rehabilitation in order to: (1) optimize their functioning within the constraints placed on them by their disease, (2) educate patient and family in reducing risk of secondary events, and (3) assist in performing activities of daily living and return to appropriate vocational status.

When designing the exercise prescription consideration should be given to the patient's stage of convalescence and individual needs. Caution and discretion should be used in prescribing the intensity of exercise. Changes in exercise intensity or changes in medications may result in signs and symptoms that may indicate an adjustment of the exercise prescription. Orthopedic and/or neuromuscular signs and symptoms may also appear which may indicate adjusting the prescription. An initial exercise prescription should be confirmed only after closely monitoring the patient's responses to the prescription. Adjustments may be required to align target heart rate and predicted exercise intensity (i.e., METs, perceived exertion, pace).

RISK STRATIFICATION

Patients with CAD vary in the severity of their atherosclerosis, amount of necrotic or ischemic myocardium, the impairment of ventricular function, and the frequency and severity of various signs or symptoms, including silent and symptomatic ischemia, dysrhythmias, abnormal blood pressure, and heart rate responses to exercise and fatigue. A careful evaluation of these various features of CAD is needed to appropriately assess the patient's prognosis for reinfarction, cardiac arrest, or heart failure and determine his/her functional capacity. Clinical decisions regarding the appropriateness for exercise training, the type and intensity of exercise to be prescribed, and the nature of medical monitoring or supervision will be determined primarily by the patient's prognosis and functional capacity.

The objective of the exercise plan for the patient with CAD is to maximize safety, efficacy, and adherence. Patient safety is paramount, thus factors influencing prognosis should be considered first. The objective of stratifying patients for cardiac rehabilitation is to determine the risk for their developing MIs, cardiac arrest, or heart failure in the near future. This risk assessment should be used to determine if more extensive cardiac evaluations are necessary, if cardiac rehabilitation, surgical or other medical treatment is indicated, and the nature of the medical supervision to be provided for exercise training. Of special interest is the likelihood that for a specific patient, exercise will induce or increase the severity of a cardiac event.

The risk for developing new clinical manifestations of CAD is primarily influenced by the extent of left ventricular dysfunction and myocardial ischemia existing at the time of evaluation. Other clinical factors to consider are the patient's age, gender, risk factor status (especially cigarette smoking), degree of atherosclerosis and possible complex or frequent cardiac dysrhythmias. During the clinical examination, evaluation of chest pain, including its type, frequency, duration and cause, provides information on ischemia. Information on myocardial damage can be obtained by history of MI, digitalis and diuretic use, chronic heart failure, left ventricular hypertrophy, cardiomegaly, rales or murmurs, ventricular gallop, Q waves, ST-segment changes, or conduction abnormalities. If patients exhibit significant left ventricular dysfunction or ischemia at rest, they are considered to be at high risk and usually are not candidates for exercise testing or exercise training.

In patients considered to be at moderate or low risk following a clinical examination, symptom-limited exercise testing can provide additional prognostic information as well as an objective measure of functional capacity. Exercise test variables that should be considered prognostic include peak exercise intensity, ability to increase systolic blood pressure, peak heart rate, angina, ST-segment displacement (especially greater than 2 mm), heart rate at onset of ischemia (angina or ST change), and ventricular dysrhythmias. Generally, the sign- and symptom-free exercise capacity is used to determine the initial exercise training intensity and target heart rates.

Additional testing to help refine the prognosis in those patients considered to be at moderate risk, based on their clinical evaluation and non-invasive exercise test, includes rest or exercise radionuclide angiography, thallium scintigraphy pre- and post-exercise, rest and exercise echocardiography, and cardiac catheterization. During these evaluations, prognostic responses include rest and exercise ejection fraction and change in ejection fraction with exercise, wall motion abnormalities, indices of ischemia (transient defects, hypoperfusion, ST changes), left ventricular end-diastolic pressure and left ventricular end-diastolic volume, and magnitude of coronary atherosclerosis. The results of these tests should be used to guide the medical management of the patient, including the nature and timing of the rehabilitation program.

Beyond just assessing the patient's functional status and general prognosis for a cardiac event, the objective of the evaluation when exercise-based rehabilitation is being considered is to evaluate his/her risk for having a cardiac event during exercise. Many of the same patient characteristics that predict general risk also predict risk during exercise. Listed in Table 6–1 are the patient characteristics found to be associated with an increased risk for cardiac events during exercise in patients with known CAD. In addition, Table 6–2 further stratifies patients according to low, intermediate, and high risk. It is important to

Table 6–1. Patient Characteristics Associated with an Increased Risk for Cardiac Events During Exercise

Clinical Status
- Multiple myocardial infarctions
- Poor left ventricular function (ejection fraction <40% at rest)
- History of chronic congestive heart failure
- Rest or unstable angina pectoris
- Complex dysrhythmias
- Left main coronary artery or three vessel atherosclerosis on angiography

Exercise Test Response
- Low exercise tolerance (<4 METs)
- Low peak heart rate off drugs (<120 beats·min^{-1})
- Severe ischemia (ST >2 mm)
- Angina pectoris at low heart rate or workload
- Inappropriate systolic blood pressure response (decrease with increasing workloads)
- Complex cardiac dysrhythmias, especially in patients with poor left ventricular function

Exercise Training Participation
- Exercises above prescribed limits

Table 6–2. Low-, Intermediate- and High-Risk Classification*

Low-risk Patients
- Following uncomplicated myocardial infarction or by-pass surgery
- Functional capacity ≥8 METs on 3-week exercise test
- Asymptomatic at rest with exercise capacity adequate for most vocational and recreational activities
- No ischemia, left ventricular dysfunction or complex dysrhythmias

Intermediate-risk Patients
- Functional capacity <8 METs on 3-week exercise test
- Shock or CHF during recent myocardial infarction (<6 months)
- Inability to self-monitor HR
- Failure to comply with exercise prescription
- Exercise-induced ischemia of <2 mm ST

High-risk Patients
- Severely depressed left ventricular function (EF <30%)
- Resting complex ventricular dysrhythmias (Lown grade IV or V)
- PVCs appearing or increasing with exercise
- Exertional hypotension (≥15 mm Hg)
- Recent myocardial infarction (<6 months) complicated by serious ventricular dysrhythmias
- Exercise-induced ischemia of >2 mm ST
- Survivors of cardiac arrest

*Health and Public Policy Committee, American College of Physicians. Cardiac Rehabilitation Services. *Ann Intern Med 15*:671–673, 1988.

consider these features in the design of each patient's rehabilitation program.

Since coronary atherosclerosis is a highly dynamic process, as is ventricular dysfunction and ischemia, a patient's prognosis and functional status is required in order to insure appropriate medical management, including rehabilitation services.

INPATIENT EXERCISE PROGRAMS (PHASE I)

The inpatient exercise program is frequently offered for the following inpatient groups: post-myocardial infarction, post-operative cardiovascular, pulmonary disease, peripheral vascular disease patients, and any others that may benefit from such services while in the hospital. The inpatient program usually includes supervised ambulatory therapy. The staff-patient ratio is generally 1:1. ECG monitoring equipment must be available for determining appropriate exercise responses and an emergency team should be available on the premises. The goals of the inpatient exercise program are to provide additional medical surveillance of patients, to return patients to activities of daily living, to offset the deleterious physiological and psychological effects of bed rest, and to prepare patients and families for stages of cardiac rehabilitation and life at home that will follow. The goals of the program should be individualized to the needs of the patient. Those patients who have been quite sedentary (e.g., some elderly patients) may require only an exercise program that allows them to return to activities of daily living (ADL). Other patients may be strong candidates for tertiary prevention activities and may begin lifelong programs to improve cardiorespiratory endurance, body composition, flexibility, and muscular strength/endurance.

INPATIENT EXERCISE PRESCRIPTION METHODS

Contraindications for inpatient participation in ambulatory exercise are given in Table 6–3. Presence or development of these special problems may require temporary delay of initiation or discontinuance of the exercise program until the appropriate medical management has alleviated the problem. The staff must be aware of the patient status daily before beginning exercise.

Termination points for an inpatient exercise session are generally more conservative than those outlined for terminating an outpatient session or exercise test (Table 6–4). Further diagnostic evaluation of the patient is warranted if any of the following signs or symptoms occur during the inpatient exercise

Table 6–3. Contraindications for Entry into Inpatient and Outpatient Exercise Programs

The following criteria may be used as contraindications for program entry.

1. Unstable angina
2. Resting systolic blood pressure >200 mm Hg or resting diastolic blood pressure >100 mm Hg
3. Orthostatic blood pressure drop of ≥20 mm Hg
4. Moderate to severe aortic stenosis
5. Acute systemic illness or fever
6. Uncontrolled atrial or ventricular dysrhythmias
7. Uncontrolled sinus tachycardia (>120 beats·min^{-1})
8. Uncontrolled congestive heart failure
9. 3° A-V heart block
10. Active pericarditis or myocarditis
11. Recent embolism
12. Thrombophlebitis
13. Resting ST displacement (>3 mm)
14. Uncontrolled diabetes
15. Orthopedic problems that would prohibit exercise

Table 6–4. Criteria for Termination of an Inpatient Exercise Session

The following guidelines may be used to terminate the exercise session for cardiac inpatients
1. Fatigue
2. Failure of monitoring equipment
3. Light-headedness, confusion, ataxia, pallor, cyanosis, dyspnea, nausea, or any peripheral circulatory insufficiency
4. Onset of angina with exercise
5. Symptomatic supraventricular tachycardia
6. ST displacement (3 mm) horizontal or downsloping from rest
7. Ventricular tachycardia (3 or more consecutive PVCs)
8. Exercise-induced left bundle branch block
9. Onset of 2° and/or 3° A-V block
10. R on T PVCs (one)
11. Frequent multifocal PVCs (30% of the complexes)
12. Exercise hypotension (>20 mm Hg drop in systolic blood pressure during exercise)
13. Excessive blood pressure rise: systolic ≥220 or diastolic ≥110 mm Hg
14. Inappropriate brachycardia (drop in heart rate greater than 10 beats·min^{-1}) with increase or no change in work load

session: increased heart rate above the prescribed limit, a marked change in blood pressure response to exercise, significant increase in shortness of breath on exertion, myocardial ischemia, significant dysrhythmias, angina pectoris, incisional pain, or excessive fatigue.

In the initial phase (1 to 3 days post-myocardial infarction or surgical procedure) of the inpatient program, activities should be restricted to low intensity (approximately 2 to 3 METs). Generally, these activities reduce risk of thrombi and consist of self-care activities and selected arm and leg exercises designed to maintain muscle tone, reduce orthostatic hypotension, and maintain joint mobility. Patients should progress with these exercises from lying to sitting and then standing. Orthostatic stress may be as important as exercise. Initial daily orthostatic stress should include unsupported standing with muscle movement for 1 to 2 minutes with blood pressure and heart rate monitoring. These activities are useful to establish response patterns for various vasodilator and beta blocking medications. Eventually (3 to 5 days post-event) walking, treadmill or cycle ergometry may be added. Although the inpatient exercise session may follow the pattern of warm-up, endurance aerobic activity, and cool-down, exercise sessions may be as short as 5 to 10 minutes per session. It is important to remember that most of the time the exercise intensity is so low and the session so short that warm-up and cool-down are not applicable. However, the patient should be informed of these procedures (use of stretching or light range of motion activities as the warm-up before the aerobic activity). As specified in Chapter 5, exercise intensity may be set as low as 40 to 60% of the patient's functional capacity. However, functional capacity of the inpatient may not be known and, in such cases, should be assumed to be quite low (3 to 5 METs).

Although heart rate may be a useful technique for prescribing exercise intensity with some inpatients, it may be impractical with others (e.g., patients with beta blocking and calcium channel blocking medications). Generally, standing resting heart rate plus 10 to 20 beats·min^{-1} or an RPE of 11 to 13 on the Borg scale is an appropriate intensity index for inpatients. For those with a functional capacity estimated or measured at 3 to 5 METs, duration might be set at 5 to 10 minutes with 2 to 4 sessions performed per day. Those with lower functional capacities may require shorter duration and more frequent sessions per day (see Chapter 5). As duration is extended, frequency of exercise can be reduced. Duration of exercise should be gradually increased to 20 to 30 minutes 1 to 2 times daily (for the length of the hospital stay) and an exercise test should be conducted prior to increasing the exercise intensity to greater than 5 METs.

DISCHARGE PLANNING

The following topics should be included in the development of the discharge plan: the patient's own personal health problems, activities of daily living, leisure time activities, appropriate rest, work, sexual activity, symptoms, and referral into a supervised Phase II rehabilitation program. At the time of discharge the patient should have information pertaining to normal coronary anatomy and his/her own disease in order for him/her to understand the alterations that occurred with atherosclerosis. Since self-care has been practiced during the period of hospitalization, personal hygiene fundamentals including bathing, toileting, dressing, and shaving should present no problem. However, instructions for the avoidance of extremes in humidity and temperature should be provided. The amount of time for appropriate rest should be specified. An afternoon nap may be suggested. When sleep is impossible, resting quietly is recommended. Knowledge of the patient's work pattern, as well as the type of work is necessary to tailor a prescription for activity (role of the vocational rehabilitation counselor). If their job entails lifting, guidance about abstaining from breath holding and the Valsalva maneuver would be appropriate as well as instruction about the number of pounds to be lifted. Most patients can resume sexual activity within 4 to 8 weeks after MI. Patients experiencing chest pain or discomfort during intercourse may be directed to take nitroglycerin before intimacy. Patients noting symptoms that include palpitation, dyspnea, angina, sleeplessness, or marked fatigue should report them to their physicians.

Near the end of the patient's time in the hospital a visit to the hospital's outpatient rehabilitation facility is recommended. If this is not possible, an informational video about the program and benefits would be an important consideration. At the time of discharge, referral forms for admittance into the rehabilitation program and an appointment for the first visit should be completed. The integration of the Phase I and II staff is important for the recruitment of new patients into the Phase II program. Continual contact with the patient by the rehabilitation staff develops confidence and enhances the patient's likelihood for beginning and adhering to the rehabilitation process.

OUTPATIENT OR HOME EXERCISE PROGRAMS (PHASE II)

Patients who have recently experienced MIs and/or coronary artery bypass surgery are at greater risk for having documented dysrhythmias. Higher incidence of angina pectoris, dysrhythmias, and dyspnea have been reported in these groups. Lightheadedness and supraventricular dysrhythmias appear more frequently in the bypass patients, whereas ST-segment changes occur more frequently in infarction patients. The higher incidence of medical problems in these patients reflect the need for monitored exercise programs.

As pointed out earlier, the comprehensive cardiac rehabilitation endeavor consists of the first few days of hospitalization (Phase I) through the early outpatient period (Phase II) and proceeds into the late outpatient (Phase III) and maintenance programs (Phase IV). The Phase II program should begin immediately after dismissal from the hospital. This would usually be the second or third week after MI or open heart surgery, and is an important time for continued medical surveillance as well as beginning intervention programs for lifestyle changes. In many instances the rehabilitation program provides an environment for group and/or individual counseling sessions about medical problems encountered and necessary lifestyle changes.

Ideally, the Phase II program should be administered on an outpatient basis in a hospital or other facility in which ECG monitoring, emergency support and direct professional supervision are available. In such programs the staff-patient ratio may vary from 1:1 to 1:5 depending on the functional capacity, symptoms and ECG characteristics of patients involved. If an outpatient program is not available or feasible, the Phase II exercise program may be implemented by the patient at home or at a community-based facility. With home programs it is preferred that the patient periodically attend an outpatient program for monitored reevaluation. Regardless of site, the goal of the Phase II rehabilitation program is to provide physical rehabilitation for resumption of habitual and occupational activities and to promote positive lifestyle changes. The program is operated under the direction of a physician who may be in attendance regularly with outpatient programs or who may be on call for home, community-based or outpatient sessions.

EXERCISE PRESCRIPTION METHODS

Exercise prescription in Phase II programs varies with the functional capacity of the patient. In general, for patients with functional capacities of 5 METs or less the techniques discussed for inpatients are appropriate. For patients with functional capacities above 5 METs the prescriptive techniques using heart rate and RPE as discussed in Chapter 5 are applicable. Frequency of exercise should be 3 to 4 sessions per week. Duration of exercise should be gradually increased from as little as 10 to 15 minutes to as much as 30 to 60 minutes as the patient's functional capacity and clinical status improve.

There are several methods used in the exercise conditioning of the cardiac patients and they include interval, circuit, circuit-interval, and continuous.

Interval Conditioning. Interval conditioning is defined as work followed by a properly prescribed relief (rest) interval. Some advantages to this form of conditioning are that each patient can (1) perform more physical work during exercise and (2) exercise at a higher intensity.

Circuit Conditioning. Circuit conditioning is explained as work performed on a number of exercise modalities with or without relief sessions between the modalities. The circuit often includes various weight lifting apparatuses for the arms and legs. A benefit of this kind of conditioning is that both arms and legs are trained.

Circuit-interval Conditioning. Circuit-interval conditioning is a combination of both circuit and interval training. The participants exercise on a number of exercise modes, while incorporating rest intervals between modes. Advantages for this type of training include those for interval and circuit conditioning.

Continuous Conditioning. In contrast to interval conditioning, continuous conditioning imposes a submaximal energy requirement that is consistent throughout the training period. These activities have been used because they are inexpensive and require little coordination for execution.

While the initial exercise prescription is based on the data (METs, heart rate, RPE, and symptoms) collected during the entrance graded exercise test, progression of patients in these programs is individualized. A reasonable progression rate is about 1 MET per 2-week interval. Each patient's prescription should be reviewed and updated with regard to intensity and duration each week.

Patients have their heart rhythm and rate monitored before, during (rhythm strips may be selected at different exercise stations), and after each exercise session. Early in the Phase II rehabilitation process rhythm monitoring may be completed by use of a single-lead electrocardiographic radiotelemetry system. This type of monitoring is helpful in observing dysrhythmias and ST-segment changes. However, during the final weeks of Phase II exercise training it seems important from a psychological point of view to wean patients from continuous monitoring. At this point strips may be obtained by use of the paddles on the defibrillator. Although strip monitoring is useful and important, blood pressure and RPE measurements are essential. These should be completed as necessary, but at a minimum blood pressure should be completed at rest, during (one leg station and one arm station) and following the cool-down period. More frequent blood pressure monitoring is required for patients who have either hypotensive or hypertensive responses to exercise.

CRITERIA FOR DISCHARGE FROM AN OUTPATIENT (PHASE II) PROGRAM

The duration of an outpatient program varies in accordance with local program guidelines. Most programs start within 1 week of hospital discharge and last between 2 and 12 weeks depending upon clinical judgment prior to entrance into a community (Phase III) program. Standard criteria for discharge from an outpatient program are not currently defined. However, the following criteria should be considered:

- Functional capacity. Since the patient's essential daily activities after hospital discharge require up to 3 METs, the patient should have a 5 MET capacity, which will allow a safe range of metabolic reserve during sustained activity of up to 3 METs.
- Medical status. The medical status of the patient should be stable. The following criteria should be met:
  - — normal hemodynamic responses to exercise including appropriate increases in blood pressure (*the ischemic threshold should be at a much greater rate-pressure product than the activity prescription*),
  - — a normal or unchanged ECG at peak exercise with normal or unchanged conduction, dysrhythmias stable or absent and a stable or medically acceptable ischemic response,
  - — angina stable or absent, and
  - — stable and/or controlled resting heart rate and blood pressure (i.e., less than 90 beats·min^{-1} and 140/90, respectively).
- Physical fitness. The patient should have an adequate level of physical fitness (i.e., muscular strength, endurance, and body composition) for daily activities and/or occupation.
- Education. Patients should have satisfactory understanding of the following:
  - — basic pathophysiology of their cardiovascular disease,
  - — rationale for the intervention approach being employed,
  - — lifestyle characteristics associated with low risk of CAD,
  - — reason(s) for any prescribed cardiovascular medications and expected side-effects, and

— range of safe activities permitted including sexual activity and vocational and recreational pursuits.

In addition, patients should demonstrate an ability to maintain the exercise prescription within the designated range and to recognize signs and symptoms of exertional intolerance.

OUTPATIENT GROUP PROGRAMS VERSUS HOME PROGRAMS

Recent research indicates that some carefully screened cardiac patients are candidates for home exercise training programs, but most authorities recommend that cardiac patients, at least initially, exercise in a group setting under medical supervision. A medically supervised outpatient rehabilitation program has distinct advantages, including close patient surveillance, expert assistance in progressing through the activity program, availability of patient education services, and social support to facilitate patient adherence to the prescribed regimen. However, many patients do not have or take the opportunity to enroll in supervised rehabilitation programs due to lack of program availability, financial situation, or other concerns. Home activity programs are feasible and beneficial for many low-risk cardiac patients, and after careful screening, even higher risk coronary patients may exercise at home. Patient surveillance of home exercise can be accomplished by a variety of means: periodic rehabilitation clinic visits, periodic primary physician visits, transtelephonic ECG transmission, and self monitoring. The mode of activity for home exercise could include walking, jogging, bicycling, swimming, cycle ergometry, rowing ergometers, exercise video tapes, etc. It is of paramount importance that family members be instructed in CPR in order to minimize risk. In addition, for patients referred to a rehabilitation center, gradual weaning to home exercise is critical in order to minimize potential patient perceived dependence on physical activity supervision.

Group programs offer advantages for patient teaching and instruction, promote compliance with the overall medical program, and permit validation of the exercise prescription and verification of the patient's ability to implement the exercise program safely and effectively. Finally, group programs may also serve to provide psychosocial support, promote understanding of the disease and its treatment, and reduce patient anxiety and depression.

Adherence is another issue when considering the recommendation of group versus home exercise programs. Many individuals prefer group over individual exercise. Social reinforcement through camaraderie and companionship found in a group program may enhance exercise adherence.

COMMUNITY EXERCISE PROGRAMS (PHASE III)

Participants in community exercise programs may have progressed through hospital inpatient and outpatient programs or may have been referred without previous participation. These programs may accept patients with various cardiorespiratory problems. As a general rule, community-based exercise programs include patients who are approximately 6 to 12 weeks post-hospital discharge, have clinically stable or decreasing angina, medically controlled dysrhythmias during exercise, a knowledge of symptoms, and the ability to self-regulate their exercise. Frequently, pulmonary patients and those with inadequately controlled hypertension may benefit from such programs. Admission criteria vary and must be based on clinical and policy judgments. The community program provides an on-going plan in which patients may exercise indefinitely. The suggested minimum functional capacity of participants for entry into the community program is 5 METs, but patients with a lower MET capacity may be admitted with increased surveillance depending on local circumstances. Phase III programs need not be located in a clinical setting and may be offered three or more times per week.

An effective community program requires a minimum of two qualified staff members (e.g., ACSM-certified Exercise Specialists or Program Directors) standing orders for emergency procedures, emergency equipment, an on-call emergency team, and a staff-patient ratio of not greater than 1:10. All staff should be trained in CPR. Electrocardiographic monitoring can be performed in a community setting, but this is not typical and may require additional staff and equipment. Spot checks of rhythms with defibrillator paddles may suffice in most cases.

Efforts should be made to move participants gradually to programs with less supervision. Participants who prove that they can self-regulate their exercise programs should be given increased freedom to do so. The frequency of follow-up exercise testing and medical evaluation is up to the patient's primary physician. However, regular medical follow-up and exercise testing is essential (i.e., 3 to 6 month basis and eventually on an annual basis or as needed).

EXERCISE PRESCRIPTION METHODS

Since most participants in community exercise programs have functional capacities greater than 5 METs, the exercise prescription methods described in Chapter 5 are usually applicable. During the first 3 to 6 months of participation the patient's exercise prescription should be gradually increased up to a duration of 45 minutes or more at 50 to 85% of functional capacity, 3 to 4 sessions per week. Exercise intensity should be based on the patient's clinical status and pathological abnormalities. After the desired functional capacity has been attained (usually 8 METs or more), maintenance should be the principal goal of the community exercise program which means no further increase in duration. However, the patient may be able to exercise consistently at a higher intensity of exercise.

Primary concerns of community programs should be promotion of adherence with the exercise prescription and other behavior modification goals. Since the ultimate goal for patients is lifelong exercise participation and because patients often remain in community programs for many months, special attention and emphasis must be placed on patient motivation. Projects such as mileage charts and weight loss lotteries are effective in enhancing motivation. Incorporation of various exercise modalities and recreational activities in addition to the formal exercise prescription may assist the participant in adhering to lifelong physical activity.

CRITERIA FOR DISCHARGE FROM A COMMUNITY PROGRAM

The duration of a community program varies depending upon local program guidelines, but most programs start 6 to 12 weeks after hospital discharge and last 6 to 12 months (some patients who do not meet the criteria for discharge may stay in these programs indefinitely). These programs may or may not be preceded by a Phase II outpatient program. There is no consensus on standard criteria for discharge for a community program, but suggested criteria are similar to those proposed for discharge from an outpatient program as outlined above:

- Functional capacity. After 3 to 12 months of participation in a community program a higher functional capacity may result. With higher risk patients and/or those with multiple medical complications, functional capacity changes may be minimal. Since most vocational and recreational activities have a wide variance, the expected functional capacity goals should be consistent with vocational and recreational requirements/goals of the individual. A careful interview and possible work evaluation to assess or evaluate responses to actual work activities should yield the necessary information for making this decision on an individual basis. At the very least, a 5 MET capacity would allow a safe range of metabolic reserve for most of the necessary daily activities.

- Medical status. The same criteria established above for the patient being discharged from a Phase II program can be applied here.
- Physical fitness. The criteria for discharge of a Phase II patient apply here as well. It should be anticipated that the patient who has participated in an extended community program will have a greater functional reserve, and will be more likely to be interested in activities with a higher metabolic demand.
- Education. The criteria outlined for the behavioral lifestyle intervention characteristics of the patient being discharged from a Phase II program can also be used for the Phase III patient. However, it should be emphasized that the Phase III patients will have participated for a greater length of time and presumably will have received more frequent evaluation in order to monitor progress and provide feedback. Specific mechanisms of follow-up evaluation need to be incorporated in order to modify the intervention plan if necessary and ensure that the behavioral objectives are being met.

RESISTIVE TRAINING GUIDELINES

The responses to resistive exercise training are different than those of dynamic exercise training (see Chapter 2). In general, patients with good left ventricular function respond to isometric exercise similarly to those with no cardiac problems. Isometric work may result in left ventricular decompensation in patients with poor left ventricular function. Therefore, it is important to minimize pure isometric work. For most patients, however, resistive training, which involves a significant dynamic work component, is often desirable to maintain and improve muscle strength and prepare patients for many vocational and recreational activities. Exclusion criteria for resistive training include: abnormal hemodynamic responses or ischemic changes on the electrocardiogram during graded exercise; patients with poor left ventricular function; peak exercise capacity <6 METs; uncontrolled hypertension or dysrhythmias. Low level resistance training may be initiated as early as 7 to 8 weeks post-event as long as a symptom-limited exercise test has been performed. The patient should be exercising in a supervised setting. The information obtained from a symptom-limited exercise test may be used to determine limits for resistive training. Although a target heart rate range may be used as a part of the guidelines for intensity during resistive training, the rate-pressure product (RPP) may be a better indicator. Resistive training will result in an increased RPP, primarily through a higher systolic pressure, with lesser contribution of heart rate. Therefore, periodic monitoring of the RPP may be important to ensure that patients do not exceed the RPP at which symptoms or electrocardiographic changes indicative of ischemia occurred during exercise testing. This can be accomplished by monitoring heart rate and arm blood pressure during resistive leg training. During arm exercise blood pressure measurements can be obtained by measuring ankle pressures or having the patient perform the exercise with a blood pressure cuff ready to be inflated. It is also possible to have the patient continue the exercise with one arm and take the blood pressure quickly in the other arm. Blood pressures measured with arterial lines during isometric exercise have shown that blood pressure drops dramatically within the first seconds after release of the effort. Therefore, cuff pressures taken immediately after resistive exercise will not reflect the pressures during the effort.

Setting an initial weight is often difficult, and may be done in any of the following ways. Forty percent of the weight obtained during one-repetition maximum for each exercise may be used as the starting weight. A more conservative approach would be to determine the weight that can be lifted only 3 times by the patient. This weight has been estimated to be 90% of maximal. Forty percent of this weight may be used as the starting weight. Another prudent method would be to start with the lowest weight on the machines and monitor responses during 10 repetitions. If the patient is well below target heart rate, RPP, and tolerates that weight well, then the weight may be increased to the next level. Titration of the weight in this manner may provide the rehabilitation supervisor with valuable information about the responses of each patient to the resistive training. Each patient should work up to 3 sets of such exercise, with the set consisting of 12 to 15 repetitions in 30 seconds with 30 seconds rest between each exercise.

Proper orientation of each patient to the exercise regimen is essential, including body position, speed and range of movement at each station, proper breathing patterns and avoidance of the Valsalva maneuver.

SPECIAL CONSIDERATIONS

ANGINA PECTORIS

Patients with stable angina pectoris for whom bypass or PTCA is not appropriate and/or those with a high (4 METs or greater) angina threshold are candidates for exercise programs. However, in those patients with angina pectoris thresholds of 2 to 3 METs, exercise may not be appropriate. A primary goal of physical conditioning in the patient with angina pectoris is to increase the amount of exercise performed before the onset of limiting angina pectoris. The patient must be evaluated for ischemic responses before, during, and after the exercise test. An essential element of this evaluation is the patient's description of the anginal episodes. This evaluation should include: (a) verbal description of symptoms (e.g., discomfort, pressure, tightness, burning, shortness of breath); (b) location of symptoms (e.g., substernal, jaw, teeth, throat, interscapular area, elbow, arm, wrist, epigastrium); (c) observed actions of the patient (e.g., clenched fist, rubbing); (d) duration and frequency of the episodes; (e) precipitating and resolving factors (e.g., exercise, rest, nitroglycerin). In evaluating the angina patient, consideration should be given to severity of disease, masking of symptoms by medications and abnormal blood pressure responses during exercise. Palpation of the painful chest area may help in differentiating musculoskeletal chest pain from that of the true angina. Teaching the patient to grade the angina symptom during the exercise test may be beneficial in determining the intensity of the discomfort for test and/or exercise session termination (+3) and to judge exertion end points (+2) during an exercise session (see Chapter 4).

Exercise Prescription Methods

Exercise intensity for angina patients should be set safely below (10 to 15 beats·min^{-1}) the ischemic threshold. This intensity combined with the frequency and duration as described in Chapter 5 may elicit the same conditioning responses or it may only prevent deconditioning. Any ischemic, dysrhythmic, and anginal response noted at the conditioning intensities should be noted in the exercise prescription.

For the patient with angina, the exercise session would include a prolonged warm-up of at least 10 minutes' duration and consist of range of motion and stretching activities. After the warm-up, the aerobic phase of the exercise session can begin (note—the aerobic phase may not be at a higher intensity than the warm-up). Patients with angina may benefit from intermittent exercise (alternating work and rest). This may be followed until the patient has sufficient strength and stamina to sustain continuous exercise. Efforts should be made to utilize all major muscle groups, including the upper extremities with dynamic repetitive motions. Breathing should be emphasized to minimize the tendency towards breath-holding. If angina occurs with exercise, the exercise period should be discontinued or at least decreased in intensity until resolved. Cool-down should be gradual and prolonged (at least 10 minutes) to prevent complications created by blood pooling in the lower extremities. Adverse hypotensive responses may occur in patients taking prophylactic nitroglycerin, especially if they are taking other antihypertensive agents (e.g., beta blockers, diuretics). Blood pressure should be checked before the use of nitroglycerin and frequently post-exercise to evaluate post-exercise hypotension. If angina is experienced with increased intensity during exercise and is not relieved by termination of exercise or by the use of three sublingual nitroglycerin tablets (one taken every 5 minutes), the patient should be transported to the nearest hospital emergency room.

PERCUTANEOUS TRANSLUMINAL CORONARY ANGIOPLASTY

Increasing numbers of patients who have had PTCA are being enrolled in all phases of cardiac rehabilitation programming. Many of these patients have had the PTCA procedure performed immediately following interruption of an acute MI with one of the available clot dissolving drugs. In addition, a number of these patients have documented severe CAD as indicated by having had dilations of multiple coronary lesions. PTCA patients are known to have a significant rate of early restenosis (23 to 30%) of the dilated vessel(s) during the first 5 to 6 months following the initial procedure. It has become apparent that close observation and monitoring of PTCA patents can detect the often rapid recurrence of hemodynamically significant restenosis in the previously dilated vessel. Thus, close monitoring during this critical time presents an interesting challenge to the cardiac rehabilitation program staff.

Exercise Prescription Methods

The previously discussed general principles of exercise prescription for cardiac patients apply to the PTCA patient. If the PTCA patient has suffered an acute MI, special precautions relating to the MI patient should also be followed. Any precautions that relate to particular medications must be considered. The PTCA patient may be on any of the common cardiac medications, but a calcium channel blocker (nifedipine, diltiazem, verapamil) and the "platelet inhibitor" drugs (dipyridamole and aspirin) are typical medications for this group of patients. The PTCA patient should be started in a medically supervised Phase I program and then progress as appropriate through Phases II and III. Ideally the Phase II program should begin in a medical facility or other setting where ECG monitoring and professional supervision is available. If the medically supervised setting is not available, a prescribed home-based exercise program may be followed. If a home-based program is necessary, it is desirable to have periodic ECG monitored reevaluations and exercise prescription updates.

The supervised cardiac rehabilitation setting for the PTCA patient can provide important surveillance for the referring physicians and can lead to the detection of the possible restenosis of the dilated vessel(s) at the site of the previous PTCA. Signs and/or symptoms may appear during an exercise session which follow several days or weeks of completely normal responses. This rather rapid onset of signs/symptoms represents restenosis of the initially dilated vessel(s) as opposed to more slowly developing progression of coronary lesions. The restenosis is detected by close observation along with appropriate ECG monitoring (Phase II setting), or close observation with subsequent quick-check monitoring of the ECG (i.e., defibrillator paddles) when symptoms are reported (late Phase II and Phase III). It is important to recognize that patients may demonstrate one of the possible combinations of diagnostic findings: (1) reported symptoms with supporting ST-segment changes on the exercise ECG, (2) reported symptoms without supporting ST-segment changes on the exercise ECG, or (3) no reported symptoms with ST-segment changes observed during exercise training.

It is essential to have well-trained exercise program staff who regularly ask the patients important questions and appropriately identify any abnormal signs/symptoms associated with possible restenosis of the dilated vessel. Important questions to ask in this patient group include: (1) How are you feeling?, (2) Have you been having any symptoms like those that you had before your angioplasty (emphasis on the location and the general quality of the pain or discomfort)?, (3) Are you having any chest discomfort with your home activities or exercise program?, and (4) Have you used any nitroglycerin at home?

PATIENTS WITH PACEMAKERS

Graded exercise testing and exercise prescription for patients with permanent pacemakers require an understanding of not only the medical status of the patient, but also the type and specific programming parameters of the pacemaker itself. Pacemakers are implanted to help manage conduction or rhythm disturbances that may occur in conjunction with, or independent of other forms of cardiovascular, pulmonary, or metabolic disease. The majority of pacemakers are employed to manage bradydysrhythmias, however, newer pacemakers and implantable defibrillators are designed to manage tachydysrhythmias.

A pacing system consists of a pulse generator and one or more leads. The pulse generator consists of the electronic circuitry and a battery. The pulse generator is surgically implanted into a subcutaneous pouch in the pectoral or abdominal area. Endocardial leads are commonly placed using a central venous approach with the subclavian vein the most frequent route used. The electrode end of the lead wire may be positioned in the right atrium, right ventricle or both so that the electrode is in contact with endocardial tissue. The lead wire is connected to the pulse generator to complete the circuit. This allows the pulse generator to sense electrical activity (both intrinsic and extrinsic) in the heart as well as to stimulate the heart according to the pacemaker type and program parameters.

To describe basic pacemaker function, a standard international five letter code (NBG) has been adopted. Pacemakers are categorized by these codes (e.g., AAI, VVI, DDD, VVIR, and AATOP) (Table 6–5). The first letter position describes the chamber(s) paced, the second letter position describes the chamber sensed, and the third letter position describes the response of the pacemaker to a sensed event. The fourth letter describes the programmability or rate modulation feature and the fifth position denotes any antitachydysrhythmia function of the pacemaker. The fourth and fifth letter codes refer to specific features and may not be employed in the coding of all pacemakers.

The most common type of implanted pacemaker is a VVI pacemaker. This pacemaker paces the right ventricle, senses electrical activity in the right ventricle and responds to sensed ventricular activity by inhibiting the pulse generator output. This type of pacemaker is most beneficial in managing ventricular bradycardias resulting from high grade AV block or sinus node exit blocks. The limitations of VVI pacing include the lack of AV synchronization and the lack of atrial contribution to cardiac output. However, with patients having complete AV block and who are pacer dependent, ventricular chronotropic response is lost despite an adequate atrial response. Under these conditions, the pacemaker is unable to pace the ventricles faster than the pacemaker's programmed rate. Therefore, the major contributing factor for increased cardiac output during activity is lost and functional capacity may be severely limited.

For patients with adequate sinus node function but high grade AV block, the DDD pacemaker offers pacing and sensing in both the atrium and ventricle. The function of the pulse generator is either inhibited or triggered by a sensed event. The DDD pacemaker offers the advantage of AV synchrony as well as rate responsiveness in patients who have appropriate SA node function with activity.

Patients who exhibit significant sinus chronotropic incompetence to exercise do not receive optimal benefits from VVI or DDD pacing during activity. However, rate responsiveness can be achieved in these patients with VVIR or DDDR pacing. For this pacing modality, the pacing rate is determined by phys-

Table 6–5. NBG Pacemaker Code

Position	*I*	*II*	*III*	*IV*	*V*
Category	*Chamber(s) Paced*	*Chambers Sensed*	*Response to Sensing*	*Programability/ Modulation*	*Antitachyarrhythmia Functioning*
	O = None	O = None	O = None	O = None	O = None
	A = Atrium	A = Atrium	T = Triggered	P = Simple Programmable	P = Pacing (Antitachyarrhythmia)
	V = Ventricle	V = Ventricle	I = Inhibited	M = Multiprogram	S = Shock
	D = Dual (A&V)	D = Dual (A&V)	D = Dual (T&I)	C = Communicating	D = Dual (P&S)
				R = Rate Modulation	

iological variables other than atrial rate. VVIR pacing provides rate responsiveness to activity, but does not allow AV synchrony and should provide the greatest opportunity for improving cardiac output during activity in appropriately selected patients. Optimal programming of rate responsive pacemakers requires a sound understanding of exercise physiology, the patient's underlying medical condition, as well as the pacemaker function. Graded exercise testing is extremely valuable to assist with the programming of rate responsive pacemakers.

All rate response sensors have relative advantages and disadvantages. The type of sensor, the mode of exercise, as well as the pacemaker programming parameters will significantly alter pacemaker responses to activity. This is especially true for non-physiological sensors such as the motion sensitive piezoelectric crystal devices. These units may function well during level treadmill activity, but can pace at an inappropriately slower rate during cycle activity or uphill walking of matched metabolic demand and over-pace during upper extremity activity of matched oxygen demand.

Antitachycardia pacemakers and automatic implantable cardioverter defibrillators (AICDs) are available to help manage tachydysrhythmia (usually with burst pacing or shock). Exercise testing and conditioning may be appropriate in these patients if activity does not provoke or aggravate the tachydysrhythmia. However, exercise testing and activity intervention pose unique problems for patients whose exercise sinus rates exceed the programmed threshold levels to activate the antitachycardia or defibrillator algorithm. Programmed activity thresholds must be noted prior to exercise testing and the protocol and/or exercise session should be terminated at a heart rate low enough to prevent device activation (appropriate programming of antitachycardia devices requires knowledge of both the peak sinus rate as well as the rate of the tachydysrhythmia).

Exercise Prescription Methods

Exercise prescriptions for patients with pacemakers should be based on treadmill test results and modified according to pacemaker response, blood pressure results, RPE, and symptom development. Pacemaker-dependent patients demonstrate a non-linear relationship between metabolism and chronotropy. Therefore, the use of standard exercise heart rate formulas in these patients is inappropriate. Instead, target MET levels or upper heart rate limits (i.e., 12 beats below upper tracking rate) are beneficial to set activity guidelines. If an accurate functional assessment is critical, the patient should undergo metabolic exercise testing.

Patients with pacemakers can engage in most conditioning activities that are appropriate for their functional capacity, symptoms, pacer response, and underlying heart disease. Although vigorous and/or ballistic upper body activities are not advised for patients with pacemakers, most physicians permit routine upper body activity. If pacemaker function is adequate and appropriate, the patient's underlying disease and symptoms, as well as their understanding of exercise principles will determine the extent of monitoring and supervision required. If the pacemaker function is inappropriate or inadequate, these issues must be resolved before formal activity is prescribed.

Exercise Testing

Reasons for exercise testing in the patient with a pacemaker include: (1) evaluation of pacemaker function, (2) evaluation of signs and/or symptoms of CAD, (3) evaluation of signs and/or symptoms of dysrhythmias, (4) pacer programming/reprogramming, (5) assessment of functional capacity, and (6) exercise prescription. Prior to performing a graded exercise test it is essential that the clinician understand the clinical question to be evaluated, the patient's clinical status (including left ventricular function, valvular, congenital, and CAD), the pacemaker type, function and current settings, as well as any activity-induced symptoms reported by the patient. Throughout the graded exercise test, close attention should be paid to symptoms, heart rate, RPE, and blood pressure response. Rhythm strips documenting changes in pacer function and/or paced complex morphology are essential. If the patient is pacemaker dependent, the ST-segments will not reflect ischemic changes. If the exercise test is being conducted to evaluate CAD, thallium or other diagnostic studies for ischemia should be considered. The clinician should also be aware that exercise blood pressure responses are often atypical in the pacemaker patient. Systolic blood pressures may rise, plateau, or fall during activity. The blood pressure response must be analyzed in conjunction with the patient's symptoms, the pacemaker function, and the clinical setting to determine the significance of the response.

Rate responsive pacemakers are designed to offer improved chronotropic response using nonatrial sensors. The magnitude and rate of chronotropic response to activity are controlled by the pacemaker's programmed parameters. Improved chronotropic response has the potential to augment functional capacity through a positive impact on cardiac output. However, patients with CAD may experience angina with improved chronotropic response secondary to increased myocardial oxygen demand. Therefore, it is essential that the clinician be aware of the patients' underlying medical status, because patients with poor left ventricular function may experience pump failure or aggravated ventricular dsyrhythmias when they are provided improved chronotropic response.

Appropriate protocol selection is critical for the pacemaker dependent patient. Most patients have low functional capacities. To assess accurately functional capacity and pacemaker function a test protocol that begins at a low MET level and increases in approximately one MET increments every 2 to 3 minutes is recommended (i.e., Naughton). Before testing a patient with an AICD, the clinician should know the threshold rate for the device. To avoid accidental discharge, the exercise test should be terminated 15 to 20 beats below threshold levels for the device (AICDs pose no hazard to clinicians in direct contact with the patient during device discharge and if required, external defibrillation can be performed without additional risk for the patient or the AICD device).

CARDIAC TRANSPLANTATION

The quality of life of the transplant patient is enhanced with an individually designed and supervised comprehensive rehabilitation program. As a result of the surgical procedure, the ventricle is no longer innervated by the autonomic system. Denervation results in a loss of autonomic modulation of cardiac output. The resting heart rate approximates the inherent rate of the sino-atrial node (100 contractions·min^{-1}). Subsequently, the cardiovascular response of the denervated heart to exercise is different. In the initial stages of exercise, enhanced venous return results in an augmented stroke volume and is responsible for an increase in cardiac output. Further elevations of cardiac output with continued exercise are a result of increases in heart rate and stroke volume resulting from circulating catecholamines. Transplant patients fail to yield the same submaximal or maximal exercise heart rate responses seen in the intact cardiovascular system (Table 6–6).

Exercise Prescription Methods

Exercise prescription for the transplant patient should incorporate the following concepts: (1) 60 to 70% of the maximal METs, (2) RPE, (3) use of the dyspnea scale, (4) longer warm-up and cool-down, and (5) the progression is individualized according to exercise tolerance. Since the heart rate response is abnormal and does not adjust with exercise intensity, the MET procedure for development of the exercise prescription will give you a workload from which to start. This workload can be fine-tuned by use of the RPE and dyspnea scales. Blood pressure should be carefully monitored at rest and during the exercise session since hypertension is a common side-effect of cyclosporin (a drug commonly administered after transplant). Abnormal exercise blood pressure responses may help identify right-sided heart failure, which may be an indication of rejection. Longer periods of warm-up and cool-down are indicated because the physiological responses to exercise and recovery take longer. Since many cardiac transplant patients have many of the same characteristics of other cardiac patients such as altered peripheral circulation and skeletal muscle metabolism, the progression of intensity, frequency and duration of exercise should be based on the patient's individual response.

Exercise personnel should be aware of the side effects of the immunosuppressive drug regimen that cardiac transplant patients must follow. Cyclosporin causes hypertension in most transplant patients, but in addition, prednisone therapy may

Table 6–6. Physiological Parameters to Consider When Prescribing and Leading Exercise or Performing Graded Exercise Tests for Cardiac Transplant Patients

1. Resting sinus tachycardia (90 to 100 contractions·min^{-1})
2. Reduced peak heart rate and delayed recovery of heart rate
3. Elevated blood pressures (a common side effect of the immunosuppressive drug regimen for most transplant patients)
4. An early onset of anaerobiosis due to a limited aerobic capacity
5. A delayed heart rate and stroke volume response
6. A diminished maximal capacity due to a reduced cardiac output
7. Absence of anginal symptoms due to denervation
8. Cardiac biopsy scores (rejection can negatively effect performance)
9. Two separate P waves may be seen on the ECG

produce the following side effects: (1) sodium and fluid retention, (2) loss of muscle mass, (3) glucose intolerance/diabetes mellitus, (4) osteoporosis, (5) fat redistribution from extremities to torso, (6) gastric irritation, (7) increased appetite, (8) increased susceptibility to infection, (9) predisposition to peptic ulcers, and (10) increased potassium excretion (see exercise in organ transplants, Chapter 7). Finally, knowledge of the most recent cardiac biopsy score is important since rejection will result in decreased exercise tolerance. If significant evidence of rejection is present, the prescribed exercise should be stopped until this is reversed.

Preliminary research on the chronic effects of exercise training in cardiac transplant patients indicates an increase in lean tissue, peak oxygen uptake, and peak heart rates. In addition, following exercise training resting blood pressure, submaximal exercise blood pressure, resting heart rate and submaximal heart rate may be reduced while maximal heart rate is increased.

CHRONIC HEART FAILURE

Patients with chronic heart failure (CHF) have limited exercise capacity that is generally a result of ventricular dysfunction and restricted cardiac output. During upright exercise there is a reduction in stroke volume reserve impairing cardiac output. Additional factors which limit exercise capacity include: (1) impairment of skeletal muscle vasodilator capacity due to chronic elevation of neurohumoral mediators of vasoconstriction, (2) decreased skeletal muscle aerobic metabolic capacity from chronic inactivity, and (3) increased pulmonary pressure.

During the initial development of cardiac rehabilitation guidelines, exercise training for CHF patients was not advised because of the potential complications of exercise stress. In addition, available medical therapy for CHF was limited to digoxin and diuretics, so that optimum treatment was seldom attained. Recent studies using invasive hemodynamic monitoring have confirmed that graduated exercise training may result in a significant improvement in peak $\dot{V}O_2$ and a decrease in heart rate response at standard exercise intensities. In addition, the maximum $a-\bar{v}O_2$ difference is increased, while arterial lactate and ventilatory threshold are reduced during exercise at a constant workload when compared to pretraining control measurements. Some patients also show an increase in maximal cardiac output. A consistent finding in all available studies is a lack of association between exercise training responses and measurements of resting left ventricular performance. This observation emphasizes the important role of peripheral adaptation mechanisms in exercise training.

CHF patients who are selected for exercise training should be stable on medical therapy and have an exercise capacity greater than 3 METs. If possible, $\dot{V}O_2$ should be determined by direct measurements since the estimation of functional capacity from treadmill exercise time in CHF patients may be erroneous. Resting left ventricular ejection fraction should be greater than 20%, although lower values are not an absolute contraindication to exercise training. The absence of exercise-induced ischemia and dysrhythmias are probably more important criteria for patient selection, because patients with these findings have a poor prognosis.

Exercise Prescription Methods

Exercise training programs for CHF patients should begin with moderate intensity (40 to 60% $\dot{V}O_{2max}$) exercise for intervals of 2 to 6 minutes separated by 1 to 2 minutes of rest. RPE ratings of 12 to 14 (on the 6 to 20 scale) are a useful guide. Training intensity and duration should be gradually increased in accordance with response to exercise and severity of heart failure. Since heart rate response may be impaired, the sensitivity of heart rate as a measure of exercise intensity is reduced and the importance of RPE is increased. ECG and blood pressure monitoring become more important to identify patients with exercise-induced dysrhythmias and hypotensive responses during and after exercise.

Potential exercise-induced complications in CHF patients include dysrhythmias and hypotension. Most patients with CHF are treated with digoxin and aggressive diuretic therapy. Hypokalemia and hypomagnesemia commonly result from chronic diuretic therapy. The combination of digoxin and altered electrolytes may precipitate malignant ventricular dysrhythmias, which are the most common cause of sudden death in CHF patients. There is always a potential for exercise training to aggravate CHF. Patients who show intolerance to exercise training or who require increasing medication are poor candidates for a training program and should be reevaluated.

MEDICATIONS AFFECTING EXERCISE TESTING AND TRAINING

Patients undergoing exercise testing and training frequently are prescribed one or more medications for management of their cardiovascular and/or other medical conditions. Many of these medications may have an impact on cardiorespiratory and/or metabolic responses to exercise. Thus, it is imperative that the health care professional be fully informed of the patient's medication regimen at the time of the exercise test, and any alteration in the medication regimen occurring prior to or during the development of the exercise prescription and exercise training.

While exercise testing for diagnostic purposes may require that a patient temporarily discontinue a medication regimen, exercise testing for the purposes of exercise prescription and training is best carried out with the patient taking his/her their prescribed drug regimen. Major additions or deletions of medications need to be taken into account during the exercise training program. Although it is desirable to have a new exercise test for appropriate alteration of the exercise prescription, this may not always be possible. An alternative would be to closely monitor the next several exercise sessions, and find an appropriate target heart rate range using the dyspnea, angina, and RPE scales.

The medications most commonly encountered in patients involved with exercise programs and their physiological effects are listed in Appendix B. These medications include those used in the control of angina, elevated blood pressure, CHF, dysrhythmias, bronchospasm, and elevated blood lipids. Among the cardiac drugs, beta blockers have the greatest effect on exercise prescription. Calcium channel blockers, nitrates and other vasodilators may alter heart rate, blood pressure and anginal threshold. Digitalis and anti-arrhythmics have few effects on exercise prescription.

BETA BLOCKERS

This class of drugs competitively inhibits the beta adrenergic receptors throughout the body. Essentially two types of beta receptors exist: the $beta_1$ and $beta_2$ receptors. The $beta_1$ receptor mediates cardiac stimulation, while the $beta_2$ receptors produce relaxation of the vascular and bronchial smooth muscle. The earliest beta blocking medication (propranolol) blocked $beta_1$

and $beta_2$ receptors. Many subsequent beta blocking agents are relatively "selective," and exert a greater effect on $beta_1$ receptors than on $beta_2$ receptors. This results in less bronchospasm, peripheral vasoconstriction and other undesirable side effects. Atenolol and metoprolol are "cardioselective" beta blockers.

Present data from clinical trials using beta blockers in post MI patients show reduced rate of reinfarction and sudden death by 20 to 25%. Beta blockers lower resting and exercise heart rate and blood pressure. Exercise heart rate is reduced at any given exercise intensity. In patients with exertional angina pectoris, beta blockers usually allow a higher achieved workload through their effect of reducing myocardial oxygen demand by lowering heart rate and blood pressure. Beta blockers may substantially lower peak workload when used in patients with severe left ventricular dysfunction due to the negative inotropic effects. Beta blockers may also precipitate or worsen CHF by diminishing myocardial contractility.

Recently developed beta blockers that have intrinsic sympathomimetic activity and provide some modest sympathetic stimulation include acebutolol and pindolol. The actions of these medications offset the decline in resting heart rate (but not maximal heart rate) commonly seen with the usual beta blockers. Another newly developed antihypertensive medication is labetolol, which has both alpha and beta blocking effects and slows heart rate while at the same time producing peripheral arterial vasodilation.

Beta blockers vary with respect to duration of action (the time during which pharmacological therapeutic effects are present). Exercise sessions performed several hours after taking some medications will result in a higher heart rate response than exercise performed closer in time to the taking of the medication. Therefore, one must be aware of the time at which the medication is taken in relation to time of exercise testing and the exercise session.

Beta blockade therapy is usually contraindicated in patients with peripheral vascular disease and claudication, coronary artery spasm, severe CHF, sinus node disease, and those receiving insulin therapy for diabetes mellitus. Annoying side effects include fatigue, depression, impotence, distinct or peculiar dreams, depressed high density cholesterol and increased triglyceride concentrations (these effects may be less pronounced with the cardioselective beta blockers and may be absent in those with intrinsic sympathomimetic activity). Sudden removal of these medications may cause angina, tachycardia, MI, sudden death, and hypertension.

In recent years, many studies have investigated the effect of beta blockers on exercise physiology and exercise training. Further research is still needed to clarify certain issues. At the present time, however, the following tentative conclusions can be drawn and recommendations made regarding beta blockers and exercise training:

1. Irrespective of the type of beta blocker prescribed, patients with CAD appear to be capable of deriving the expected improvement in cardiorespiratory fitness during exercise training;
2. In contrast to patients with myocardial ischemia, effort tolerance is generally reduced to a greater degree with nonselective beta blockers than with $beta_1$-selective blockers in physically active patients with uncomplicated essential hypertension. When possible, $beta_1$-selective blockers should therefore be used in preference to nonselective agents in patients with uncomplicated essential hypertension who lead a physically active lifestyle. However, because even $beta_1$-selective blockers may have a negative impact in certain individuals, physicians should be aware of this possible adverse effect and, if present, consider alternative therapy with drugs such as ACE inhibitors or calcium antagonists (unless beta blocker therapy is specifically indicated);
3. Intrinsic sympathomimetic activity confers no obvious advantage to hypertensive patients who engage in exercise conditioning;
4. The prescription of training heart rates for patients receiving beta blocker therapy should be based on the results of individualized graded exercise testing conducted with the patient on medication and in accordance with traditional guidelines. Ideally, graded exercise testing and training should be performed at a similar time interval after ingestion of the last drug dose when heart rate based exercise prescriptions are employed.

NITRATES

Nitrate preparations directly relax both the venous and arterial vascular systems. Venodilatation decreases the return of blood to the heart and thus diminishes preload, while arteriolar vasodilatation decreases the systemic vascular resistance thus reducing afterload. The combined effects result in reduced myocardial oxygen consumption and reduced ischemia in patients with CAD. Nitrates may improve exercise capacity by increasing the anginal threshold. The use of sublingual nitroglycerin immediately prior to exercise may eliminate or reduce the likelihood of the occurrence of angina. However, venous dilatation and diminished arterial pressure may result in hypotension particularly with the abrupt cessation of exercise. Long-acting nitrates either in oral form or applied transdermally as ointments or patches have been documented to have an antianginal benefit, particularly after a brief nitrate-free interval (6 to 8 hours daily), which prevents the development of patient nonresponsiveness, or tolerance and loss of anti-anginal efficacy. Nitrates do not directly affect the heart rate response to exercise so alteration of the exercise prescription is not necessary.

CALCIUM CHANNEL BLOCKERS

This class of drugs competitively inhibits the inward flow of calcium into cardiac and smooth muscle cells, thereby reducing vascular tone and producing vasodilatation in the coronary artery beds and in the peripheral arteries. They may also have modest negative inotropic effects and slow the rate of conduction between the atria and ventricles. Afterload is reduced, resulting in a reduction in blood pressure. Thus, the anti-anginal effect is produced by both an improved myocardial oxygen supply as well as a lower myocardial oxygen demand. The 1,4-dihydropyridine derivatives (such as nifedipine) have the most potent vasodilatory effect and can result in light-headedness and peripheral edema as well as a reflex tachycardia. These side effects are less likely with the use of verapamil and diltiazem. Nitrendipine, the newest calcium blocker to be approved, has actions similar to nifedipine.

Verapamil, and to a lesser degree, diltiazem, may show negative inotropic effects as well as a slowing of AV conduction. Therefore, caution is required when combining either of these calcium channel blockers with beta blockers. As with the beta blockers, consideration needs to be given to the exercise prescription based upon the patient's calcium channel blocker treatment. Heart rate prescription should be based on exercise tolerance test data performed with the patients taking their usual medical regimen.

DIURETICS

The overall effect of diuretics is to increase renal excretion of sodium and extracellular fluid. This produces a reduction in arteriolar sodium content and results in a decreased peripheral vascular resistance and reduction of blood pressure. The thiazide diuretics as well as the "loop" diuretics (furosemide and ethacrynic acid) may also produce a loss of potassium from the body with subsequent muscular fatigue, weakness, and the potential for ventricular irritability. Although diuretics have no effect on heart rate response to exercise, the potential for hypovolemic and hypokalemic states needs to be recognized. Though the exercise prescription needs no alteration in patients using these drugs, hypokalemia may lead to a false-positive exercise ECG. Potassium-sparing diuretics, such as spironolactone and triamterene apparently do not present these problems.

VASODILATORS

This is a broad class of drugs having various mechanisms of action. Certain drugs (prazosin and terazosin) in this class produce vasodilation by means of competitive inhibition of the alpha adrenergic vasoconstricting effects in the arterial system. Other drugs (methyldopa, clonidine, guanabenz and guanfacine) suppress the central nervous system regulation of sympathetic outflow and produce vasodilation. Nonadrenergic vasodilators including hydralazine, minoxidil and pinacidil, directly produce dilation of the vascular smooth muscle. All of the drugs from this class have the potential for producing post-exercise hypotension. Allowing for adequate cool-down after an exercise session will diminish the likelihood of this effect.

ANGIOTENSIN CONVERTING ENZYME INHIBITORS (ACE INHIBITORS)

This is an emerging class of drugs (captopril, enalapril and lisinopril) that apparently reduce pressure by competitively inhibiting the conversion of angiotensin I to the potent vasoconstrictor angiotensin II. These drugs are quite effective in controlling elevated blood pressure as well as relieving the symptoms of CHF. Two clinical trials of ACE inhibitors have documented reduced mortality in patients with advanced heart failure compared with placebo treatment. These drugs tend to produce modest retention of potassium, and generally should not be combined with potassium-sparing diuretics or with potassium supplementation. They have no direct effects on the ECG and do not require modification of the exercise prescription. This class of drugs may potentiate post-exercise hypotension.

DRUG TREATMENT USED IN CHRONIC HEART FAILURE

Diuretics and ACE inhibitors are two major drug classes used for the management of CHF. In addition, digitalis preparations are frequently encountered in patients with CHF. Digitalis preparations work by limiting the sodium/potassium exchange across the myocardial cell membrane resulting in a parallel increase in sodium coupled calcium transport within the myocardial cell. This in turn results in an increased myocardial contractility. Digitalis also reduces conduction velocity through the AV node thereby reducing the rate of ventricular response to atrial fibrillation or atrial tachycardia. The effects of digitalis on the ST-segment of the electrocardiogram makes reliable interpretation of an exercise test difficult. Therefore, patients on digitalis may require other tests for assessing myocardial ischemia (i.e., thallium stress testing or persantine testing). Clinical trials have documented mild beneficial effects of digoxin preparation on exercise capacity in patients with heart failure (there is the potential for digoxin toxicity and aggravation of ventricular dysrhythmias with hypokalemia).

ANTIARRHYTHMICS

There are four classes (I–IV) of medications prescribed for the control of ventricular dysrhythmias. Class I drugs include quinidine, procainamide, disopyramide, phenytoin, tocainide, mexiletine, encainide, and flecainide. No major effects have been reported on the exercise response for the ECG and/or heart rate with the exception of quinidine and procainamide. These two drugs may cause a prolongation in the QRS and/or the QT interval. In addition, quinidine has an anticholinergic and an alpha blocking effect. Class II drugs are the beta blockers, and the current Class III drug is amiodarone. The Class IV designation is given to the calcium channel blockers. The key consideration for exercise training in patients with antiarrhythmic medications is recognition of the potential of any of these drugs to be pro-dysrhythmic (potentially increased ventricular ectopy). Furthermore, patients with significant ventricular dysrhythmias are often patients with continuing myocardial ischemia and/or CHF. Both of these classes of patients are at relatively higher risk for cardiovascular morbidity and mortality. A trial of two specific anti-dysrhythmic medications, encainide and flecainide, documented increased cardiovascular mortality and sudden death with the use of either of these drugs compared to placebo in patients having suffered an acute myocardial infarction and showing ventricular dysrhythmias. Therefore, these two drugs have a specific limitation for their use in patients with well-documented life-threatening dysrhythmias. The results of this clinical trial demonstrate the potential adverse pro-dysrhythmic effect of anti-dysrhythmic medications in patients with CAD.

BRONCHODILATORS

Theophylline drugs and sympathomimetic amines are two broad classes of medications used for bronchodilation. Theophylline drugs act by preventing or reversing bronchospasm and will have a beneficial effect in allowing a patient to engage in or continue exercise. This type of medication produces increased heart rates and may induce ventricular ectopy. The sympathomimetic agents stimulate the beta adrenergic system. Therefore, they increase heart rate and may induce hypertension as well as ventricular ectopy.

LIPID LOWERING DRUGS

Many patients with CAD as well as a large number of subjects at high risk for the development of cardiovascular disease secondary to hyperlipidemia are on various lipid lowering drugs. While none of these drugs change the exercise testing or training parameters, they are frequently encountered and the exercise specialist may be called upon to inform the patient of their mechanism of action and/or their potential side effects.

The bile acid binding resins (cholestyramine and colestipol) bind the cholesterol-rich bile acids in the intestine and cause increased loss of bile through the GI tract. In usual doses, they reduce both total and LDL cholesterol by approximately 15 to 30%. Of extreme importance to the patient who takes other medications is that bile acid binding resins also bind other medications (digoxin) and may keep other medications from being absorbed. Therefore, it is recommended that other medicines be taken at least 1 hour before or 4 hours following ingestion of bile acid binding resins. Gastrointestinal side effects are fairly common with these agents and may cause constipation.

Nicotinic acid, a water-soluble B vitamin has been shown to reduce the VLDL and LDL cholesterol and at the same time increase the HDL cholesterol levels. These changes are generally in the range of 10 to 20%, but the principal drawback is that many patients experience flushing especially at higher dose levels. This side effect is somewhat blunted by preingesting an aspirin or taking the medication at the time of a meal. Nicotinic acid can produce hepatic dysfunction or aggravate preexisting peptic ulcer or liver disease.

Lovastatin is the first of the HMG-Co A reductase inhibitor medications to be marketed. This agent competitively inhibits the HMG-Co A reductase enzyme in the liver which is the rate-limiting enzyme in cholesterol biosynthesis. These drugs can have a reasonably potent effect in lowering LDL and total cholesterol levels by 24 to 45% and at the same time enhance HDL cholesterol by approximately 10 to 15%. They do occasionally produce elevation in some liver function tests (2% of patients) and can occasionally produce myalgia (.5%). The myalgia can be fulminate in patients who are on immunosuppressive drugs (particularly cardiac and/or renal transplantation patients).

Gemfibrozil, a fibric acid derivative, inhibits the synthesis of VLDL cholesterol, which is a precursor of LDL cholesterol, and thereby reduces both triglyceride (35%) and LDL cholesterol (5 to 15%) and enhances HDL cholesterol (12%). Abnormal liver function tests are occasionally seen and this medication may aggravate the formation of gallstones and myositis.

Probucol combines with LDL cholesterol in the plasma leading to a more efficient removal of LDL from the plasma. Unfortunately, it also leads to an undesirable reduction of HDL cholesterol levels. It can produce bothersome gastrointestinal symptoms and has been shown to prolong the QT interval of the ECG.

PSYCHOTROPIC MEDICATIONS

This is a broad category of medications that include antianxiety drugs, antidepressants, and tranquilizers. The phenothiazine class of tranquilizers may increase heart rate and diminish blood pressure. They have also been reported to produce either false-positive or false-negative exercise ECG responses on rare occasions. Diazepam (Valium) may produce a modest drop in heart rate and blood pressure and may occasionally produce a false-positive exercise ECG response. Among the antidepressant medications, the tricyclics may produce reduction in blood pressure and an elevation in heart rate. They may also produce a minor increase in the PR and QT intervals and some nonspecific ST-T wave changes leading to a false-positive exercise ECG response.

NICOTINE

While not a prescribed drug, nicotine is commonly encountered in patients in cardiac exercise laboratories and exercise training programs. This class of drugs stimulates the release of epinephrine and norepinephrine resulting in an increased heart rate and elevation in blood pressure. This in turn may exacerbate angina pectoris particularly when accompanied by diminished oxygen delivering capacity due to carboxyhemoglobin accumulation from cigarette smoking. Additionally, cigarette smoking tends to reduce the HDL cholesterol levels. Ventricular ectopy can be induced by these drugs, but there is no evidence that nicotine can produce a false-positive result on an exercise ECG.

ALCOHOL

Alcohol is primarily a myocardial depressant and can cause myocardial irritability. Chronic excessive consumption can lead to a cardiomyopathy, hypertension, and manifest clinical CHF. Exercise testing within a day of excessive alcohol consumption can result in dysrhythmias (particularly atrial dysrhythmias).

REFERENCES

1. American Association of Cardiovascular and Pulmonary Rehabilitation, Position Paper: Scientific evidence of the value of cardiac rehabilitation services with emphasis on patients following myocardial infarction—Section I: Exercise conditioning component. *J Cardiopul Rehabil 10*:79–87, 1990.
2. American Heart Association: Statement on Exercise: A position statement for health professionals by the Committee on Exercise and Cardiac Rehabilitation of the Council on Clinical Cardiology, American Heart Association. *Circulation 81*:396–398, 1990.
3. DeBelder MA and Camm JA: Implantable cardioverter-defibrillators (ICD's) 1989: How close are we to the ideal device? *Clin Cardiol 12*:339–345, 1989.
4. Franklin BA, Hollingsworth V and Borysyk LM: Additional diagnostic tests:

Special populations. In *Resource Manual for Guidelines for Exercise Testing and Prescription.* Edited by American College of Sports Medicine. Philadelphia: Lea & Febiger, 1988.

5. Franklin BA, Hellerstein HK, Gordon S and Timmis GC: Cardiac patients. In *Exercise in Modern Medicine.* Baltimore: Williams & Wilkins, 1989.
6. Greenland P and Chu JS: Efficacy of cardiac rehabilitation services: With emphasis on patients after myocardial infarction. *Ann Intern Med 15*:650–663, 1988.
7. Haskell WL, Savin WM, Schroeder JS, Alderman EA, Ingles NB, Daughters GT and Stinson EB: Cardiovascular response to handgrip isometric exercise in patients following cardiac transplantation. *Circ Res* (suppl. 1), *48*:156–161, 1981.
8. Health and Public Policy Committee, American College of Physicians. Cardiac Rehabilitation Services. *Ann Intern Med 15*:671–673, 1988.
9. Kavanagh TK, Yacoub MH, Mertens DJ, Kennedy J, Campbell RB and Sawyer P: Cardiorespiratory response to exercise training after orthotopic transplantation. *Circulation 77*:162–171, 1988.
10. O'Conner GT, Buring JE, Yusuf Salim, Goldhaber SZ, Olmstead EM, Paffenbarger RS and Hennekens CH: An overview of randomized trials of rehabilitation with exercise after myocardial infarction. *Circulation 80*:234–244, 1989.
11. Oldridge NB, Guyatt GH, Fischer ME and Rimm AA: Cardiac rehabilitation after myocardial infarction. *JAMA 260*:945–950, 1988.
12. Opie LH, Chatterjee K, Gersh BJ, Harrison DC, Kaplan NM, Marcus FI, Singh BN, Sonnenblick EH and Thadani U: *Drugs for the Heart.* Philadelphia: WB Saunders, 1987.
13. Painter P and Hanson P: Isometric exercise: Implications for the cardiac patient. *Cardiovasc Rev Rep 5*:261–279, 1984.
14. Pollock ML, Pels AE, Foster C and Ward A: Exercise prescription for rehabilitation of the cardiac patient. In *Heart Disease and Rehabilitation.* Edited by ML Pollock and DH Schmidt. New York: John Wiley & Sons, 1986.
15. Sparling PB and Cantwell JD: Strength training guidelines for cardiac patients. *Phys Sportsmed 17*:190–196, 1989.
16. Sullivan MJ, Higgenbotham MD and Cobb FR: Exercise training in patients with chronic heart failure delays ventilatory anaerobic threshold and improves submaximal exercise performance. *Circulation 79*:324–329, 1989.
17. Sullivan MJ, Higgenbotham MD and Cobb FR: Exercise training in patients with severe left ventricular dysfunction; hemodynamic and metabolic effects. *Circulation 78*:506–515, 1988.
18. Superko HR: The effects of cardiac rehabilitation in permanently paced patients with third degree heart block. *J Cardiac Rehabil 3*:561–568, 1983.
19. Thompson PD: The benefits and risks of exercise training in patients with chronic coronary artery disease. *JAMA 259*:1537–1540, 1988.

CHAPTER 7

Exercise Prescription for Special Populations

The benefits of exercise training for several special populations are becoming increasingly recognized. Included in these special populations are several types of chronic disease patients. In patient groups the goals of exercise training are: (1) to counteract the detrimental physiological effects of bed rest and/or previous sedentary living patterns, and (2) to optimize the patient's functional capacity within the physiological limitations of the disease. Exercise training should be considered a part of the medical therapy because it provides a unique opportunity for surveillance and because it is a valuable source of information that may assist the physician in the ongoing treatment of the patient. In some cases the response to medical therapy becomes more evident during exercise.

For some patient populations a research-based body of knowledge on exercise testing and prescription is limited. Therefore, it is essential that exercise professionals learn as much as possible about each specific disease process and the relevant medical treatments. Such knowledge is helpful in understanding the interactions between exercise and the disease and the potential adverse effects of exercise training. Exercise therapy must not interfere with standard medical therapy and exercise testing protocols and prescription protocols must be individualized in accordance with the presence and severity of co-existing disease and treatment conditions.

The following guidelines are for exercise testing and prescription in patients with chronic diseases for which there are some published studies and significant clinical experiences. These guidelines must be used with the understanding that: (1) research is limited, and some recommendations are based on clinical experience and theoretical applications, (2) there may be patients for whom exercise is contraindicated and others who may not achieve expected physiologic changes, (3) the exercise prescription may require modification, suspension, or termination when there is a change in medical status and/or medical management, and (4) exercise should be initiated only when the patient is clinically stable.

GENERAL CONSIDERATIONS IN CHRONIC DISEASE

A primary challenge for the exercise professional who administers an exercise program for patients with chronic disease is assessing the risk/benefit relationship. Exercise testing and prescription for patients with chronic disease require individualization and also require more flexibility due to the fluctuating clinical status of patients. Patients may experience temporary set-backs, and many will have a progressively worsening course. Any significant change in medical status requires reassessment of the exercise goals and the risks associated with exercise. For example, an acute flare-up in an arthritic patient may mean that exercise could exacerbate the inflammation. Under such circumstances, it may be better to suspend exercise until the joint has improved, despite the loss of conditioning caused by the inactivity. When exercise is resumed, the original goals and prescription may have to be modified and a new risk/benefit relationship may exist.

Pain and chronic malaise are conditions that are common to many chronic disease states. The exercise professional should help the patient develop the ability to distinguish pain from the normal discomfort that is associated with vigorous exercise. RPE is a good tool for evaluating normal discomfort and should be used for regulating intensity. In contrast, pain is the body's mechanism for identifying dysfunction and injury. As such, it is a warning symptom that should never be ignored or dismissed and should be investigated before proceeding with exercise.

Exercise professionals must expect that some patients with chronic disease will have a progressively worsening course. Such circumstances may call for the discontinuation of exercise, even though major efforts and progress have been made. Perseverance is an essential part of exercise therapy, but good clinical judgment must take precedence when working with chronic disease patients.

PULMONARY DISEASE

Patients with chronic obstructive pulmonary disease (COPD) include those with emphysema, chronic bronchitis, and reactive airways disease (asthma). Abnormal pulmonary function, affecting ventilation and gas exchange, results in dyspnea upon exertion and extremely limited functional capacity. Bronchodilators and glucocorticoids are often used to open airways, expectorants are used for enhancement of mucociliary clearance, and cardioactive agents (digitalis) and diuretics are used to reduce cardiac stress in ventricular failure or cor pulmonale (pulmonary hypertension). Oxygen may be required to maintain arterial oxygen tension and counteract pulmonary hypertension. Polycythemia is usually a complicating factor, especially in smokers.

Rehabilitation for COPD patients should involve several types of professionals. Respiratory therapists evaluate, teach and assure appropriate use of bronchodilators, positive pressure breathing techniques and oxygen administration. Physical therapists may teach breathing techniques (including pursed lip breathing), assistance with expectoration, and relaxation during dyspnea. Occupational therapists may be involved to assess activities of daily living and make appropriate recommendations to reduce the oxygen requirements of the activity. Psychologists or social workers may be helpful in working with depression, fear, anxiety, hostility, denial, and sexual dysfunction that may be associated with these diseases.

All patients should be evaluated with complete pulmonary testing. Although exercise testing may be of limited diagnostic value for CAD in these patients, due to their limited functional capacity, valuable information can be gained from an exercise test. Exercise testing may aid in: (1) providing the data needed to calculate a target heart rate for exercise training; (2) determining other reasons for dyspnea and/or exercise limitations (i.e., peripheral vascular disease); (3) assessing dysrhythmias during exercise; (4) determining if oxygen may be necessary during the exercise session; and (5) determining the level of impairment that may preclude the patient from certain types of work.

Exercise testing may be done on a cycle ergometer or treadmill. The protocol must be low-level (i.e., starting at 1.5 METs and increasing 0.5 METs per stage). The protocol may be continuous or discontinuous with short durations at each stage. In addition to ECG and blood pressure monitoring, ventilation, breathing frequency, and tidal volume should be evaluated. Additional measurements such as oxygen consumption, carbon dioxide output, and arterial oxygen saturation may provide important information. Arterial blood gas analysis may be important in patients with gas exchange disturbances.

The exercise prescription must be individualized according to the patient's degree of respiratory disability as assessed by exercise and pulmonary function tests. Cycling, walking, and swimming are appropriate modes of exercise, whereas upper body exercises such as arm cranking or rowing may not be desirable because of the high ventilation required at a given power output. The mode of exercise selected should be one that is enjoyable to the patient and one that will directly improve the patient's ability to perform usual daily activities.

Exercise intensity should be prescribed according to the patient's functional capacity and limitations. Since patients with essentially normal spirometry who experience dyspnea only during heavy exertion and patients with cardiovascular disease respond to exercise training similarly, the heart rate method may be used to prescribe exercise intensity. Patients with forced vital capacity (FVC) and forced expiratory volume at 1 second (FEV_1) values between 60 to 80% of the predicted value may experience dyspnea when walking rapidly. Reductions in ventilatory capacity are not usually the limiting factors to exercise in these patients, and the exercise intensity should be maintained at the level that requires a ventilatory rate less than 75% of the patient's maximal exercise ventilation. More severely limited patients (FVC and FEV_1 <60% of the predicted value, abnormal V_D/V_T at rest and/or exercise with or without desaturation during exercise) who experience dyspnea with only mild exercise are limited by their respiratory system. Exercise intensity in these patients may be regulated by using the dyspnea scale. Some severely limited patients may require supplemental oxygen during exercise if this has been objectively demonstrated to improve exercise performance. Supplemental oxygen should be administered at high flow rates at an F_{IO_2} of 24 to 28%.

Modifications in the duration and frequency of exercise may be necessary. If a 20- to 30-minute duration of continuous exercise is an unrealistic goal, then two 10-minute sessions or four 5-minute sessions may be prescribed. Interval exercise may also be necessary until adaptations are made that enable the patient to decrease the rest intervals and gradually increase the work intervals.

Realistic expectations should be developed for COPD patients when starting an exercise training program. Most patients do not show improvements in pulmonary function, however, diligent participation can reduce respiratory symptoms, reverse anxiety and depression, and increase the ability to perform activities of daily living. Some patients may increase exercise tolerance by peripheral adaptations. Periodic evaluation of progress using a procedure such as a 12-minute walk test may be important for motivational purposes.

HYPERTENSION

Individuals with hypertension may require special considerations for exercise testing and/or prescription. Hypertension may be categorized as primary (cause unknown) or secondary (cause due to identifiable endocrine or structural disorders). Approximately 90% of hypertension is primary, and within this category there are several groups: borderline to mild hypertension (140/90), mild to moderate (150/95), moderate to severe (160/100) and uncontrolled (170/110). Individuals with chronically elevated blood pressure have an increased probability of stroke, coronary artery disease, and left ventricular hypertrophy (LVH).

Blood pressure is determined by cardiac output and the resistance to blood flow (total peripheral resistance), and therefore can be elevated either as a result of elevated cardiac output or increased total peripheral resistance, or both. Initial treatment for those with mild/borderline hypertension includes weight management, exercise and dietary restriction of sodium intake. Treatment of mild to moderate hypertension that is refractory to this approach and severe hypertension typically require medications that either lower cardiac output or peripheral resistance (see Appendix B for specific medications and their effects on the exercise response).

Dynamic exercise in mild to moderate hypertensives is accompanied by greater increases in cardiac output and systolic and diastolic blood pressure than those observed in normotensives. Severe hypertensives exhibit a drop in cardiac output due to a decrease in stroke volume and have high systolic and diastolic pressures due to significantly elevated peripheral resistance. Isometric exercise results in greater increases in both systolic and diastolic pressure in hypertensives compared with normotensives.

Standard exercise testing methods and protocols may be used for evaluation of hypertensive individuals. However, due to the high prevalence of LVH, the exercise electrocardiogram may be uninterpretable for coronary disease. Additional studies, such as thallium testing may be needed to diagnose CAD.

The frequency of exercise training should be at least 4 times per week, with daily exercise being desirable. Duration should gradually progress to 30 to 60 minutes at an intensity near the lower end of the heart rate range (40 to 65%). High intensity exercise should be discouraged. Isometric exercise is not strictly contraindicated in hypertensive patients, however, high intensity exercise and activities with a significant isometric component should be minimized in those with established hypertension. Weight training should be prescribed using low resistances and high repetitions (i.e., 20 repetitions).

The exercise prescription may have to be modified according to the prescribed antihypertensive medications. Medications that reduce total peripheral resistance by vasodilation may cause post-exercise hypotension, requiring a longer cool-down time for redistribution of blood flow. Medications that limit the cardiac output response to exercise by limiting heart rate require prescription of exercise intensity by methods other than heart rate (e.g., RPE). Patients taking diuretics for reduction of fluid volume may have low potassium levels, which may cause dysrhythmias during exercise. Some medications affect heart rate and total peripheral resistance to varying degrees. It is therefore essential that the exercise prescription be individualized and based on the heart rate and blood pressure responses to exercise testing. Any adjustment of medication requires reassessment of the patient's response to exercise and appropriate modification of the exercise prescription.

PERIPHERAL VASCULAR DISEASE

Arteriosclerosis is a common peripheral vascular disease (PVD), especially in the elderly. Other vascular insufficiencies include arterial stenosis, Raynaud's phenomenon (an abnormal vasoconstrictor reflex exacerbated by cold exposure), and Buerger's disease (an inflammation of the sheath encapsulating the neurovascular bundle in the extremities). Peripheral arteriosclerosis is associated with hypertension and hyperlipidemia, is frequently observed in patients with CAD and cerebrovascular disease, and may be seen in patients with diabetes mellitus. The advanced stages of PVD result in skin ulcerations and gangrene, which may require limb amputation.

Patients with PVD experience ischemic pain (claudication) which may be described as an aching, weakness, tightness or cramping sensation during physical activity. This pain typically is in the calf of the leg and disappears quickly upon cessation of exercise. A subjective grading of the pain can be made with the following scale:

Grade I: Definite discomfort or pain, but only of initial or modest levels (established, but minimal)

Grade II: Moderate discomfort or pain from which the patient's attention can be diverted by a number of common stimuli (e.g., conversation, interesting TV show, etc.)

Grade III: Intense pain (short of Grade IV) from which the patient's attention cannot be diverted except by catastrophic events (e.g., fire, explosion)

Grade IV: Excruciating and unbearable pain

Assessment of the extent of disease is possible through many procedures, including physical examination, Doppler studies, ankle-to-arm pressure indices, nuclear medicine flow studies, and arteriography, to name a few. Severe occlusive disease is treated initially with exercise and medications that decrease blood viscosity. Treatment with angioplasty or bypass grafting is becoming more common.

Functional capacity may be assessed using a multi-stage discontinuous protocol with the measurement of peak oxygen consumption. Testing should include subjective ratings of pain severity (Grades I to IV). Exercise testing for diagnostic purposes may require the use of arm ergometry to achieve adequate myocardial stress. Patients will be primarily limited by peripheral discomfort during treadmill or bicycle exercise.

Exercise training may result in increased symptom-limited functional capacity, perhaps through collateral vessel formation, improved distribution of blood flow, microvascular changes in the muscle and/or improved oxidative capacity in the muscle. Non-weight bearing activities may be most comfortable for the patient and often allow a longer duration and higher intensity of exercise, although walking may be more specific and result in more significant functional changes. Exercise should be performed on a daily basis incorporating intervals of intensity that elicit the maximal tolerable pain with intermittent rest/relief periods. Patients should start with 20 to 30 minutes of interval exercise twice daily and, within 4 to 6 weeks, increase the total time of the exercise to one session of 40 to 60 minutes.

As functional capacity improves with less peripheral limitation, central cardiac limitations may assume greater importance. This may require modification of the program in terms of supervision, intensity, and duration. Other lifestyle modifications should be stressed to control other contributing conditions such as glucose control, hyperlipidemia, weight control, and smoking habits.

DIABETES MELLITUS

Diabetes mellitus is a disease associated with problems in controlling blood glucose, resulting primarily in hyperglycemia. There are two types of diabetes mellitus: Type I (insulin-dependent or juvenile-onset diabetes), resulting from a pancreatic deficiency in insulin production; and Type II (non-insulin dependent or maturity-onset diabetes), usually associated with decreased cellular insulin sensitivity. Type I diabetics are dependent upon regular injections of insulin, usually given twice daily or through an infusion pump. Type II diabetics are often obese and can frequently avoid medication therapy through diet restrictions and weight loss. Type II diabetics may require oral hypoglycemic agents rather than injections of insulin. A lack of sufficient insulin results in hyperglycemia because the cellular absorption of glucose is not facilitated.

Problems associated with long-term elevation of blood glucose include microangiopathy, neuropathy (which may lead to impairment of the peripheral circulation), retinopathy, cardiovascular disease, renal disease, peripheral ulcerations, and autonomic dysfunction.

Exercise testing in diabetic patients is recommended because of the increased risk of cardiovascular disease in these patients. Low level testing protocols should be used on the treadmill or cycle ergometer. Arm ergometry may be necessary for diagnostic testing in patients who have peripheral neuropathy and/or peripheral vascular disease that impairs peripheral function. The presence of autonomic neuropathy may prevent the patient from achieving age-predicted maximal heart rates, which may reduce the sensitivity of the test.

The response to exercise in the insulin-dependent diabetic depends upon a variety of factors, including the adequacy of control with exogenous insulin. If the diabetic is under appropriate control or only slightly hyperglycemic without ketosis, exercise decreases blood glucose levels and less insulin will be required. However, problems can arise during exercise if the diabetic is not under adequate control. If there is a lack of sufficient insulin prior to exercise, glucose transport into the muscles will be impaired and glucose will not be available as an energy substrate. To compensate, free fatty acid use increases and ketone bodies are produced, possibly leading to the development of ketosis. In addition, there will be greater blood glucose production, further enhancing the hyperglycemic state. For these reasons, type I diabetics must be under adequate control prior to beginning an exercise program.

On the other hand, because exercise has an insulin-like effect, exercise-induced hypoglycemia is the most common problem experienced by exercising diabetics. Hypoglycemia may result when too much insulin is present, or if there is accelerated absorption of insulin from the injection site, which can occur with exercise. Accelerated absorption generally occurs when short-acting insulin is taken and when the injection site is near the active muscles. Hypoglycemia can occur during exercise or up to 4 to 6 hours following an exercise bout. To counteract this response, the diabetic may need to reduce insulin dosage or increase carbohydrate intake prior to exercising. Exercise programming, therefore, must include patient (and staff) education on these potential reactions.

The risk of hypoglycemic events may be minimized by taking the following precautions:

1. Monitor blood glucose frequently when initiating an exercise program
2. Decrease the insulin dose (by 1 to 2 units as prescribed by the physician) or increase carbohydrate intake (10 to 15 g per one-half hour of exercise) prior to an exercise bout
3. Inject insulin in an area such as the abdomen that is not active during exercise
4. Avoid exercise during periods of peak insulin activity

5. Eat carbohydrate snacks before and during prolonged exercise bouts
6. Be knowledgeable of the signs and symptoms of hypoglycemia
7. Exercise with a partner

Other precautions that must be taken include (1) proper footwear and practice of good foot hygiene, (2) awareness that the diabetic patient on beta-blocking medications may be unable to experience hypoglycemic symptoms and/or angina, and (3) awareness that exercise in excessive heat may cause problems due to anhydrosis.

In general, diabetics can participate in the same modes of activity as non-diabetics for their exercise training. Obese diabetics should use non-weight bearing activities to minimize risk of orthopedic injury and/or foot irritation. Daily exercise is recommended for both types of diabetics. For insulin-dependent diabetic patients, exercise should be performed daily so that a regular pattern of diet and insulin dosage can be maintained for glucose control. The non-insulin dependent diabetic should exercise at least 5 times per week to maximize caloric expenditure for the purpose of weight management.

Exercise duration is specific to the type of diabetes. Duration for the insulin-dependent diabetic may be as low as 20 to 30 minutes per session due to the higher frequency of exercise. In contrast, exercise prescription for the non-insulin dependent diabetic should maximize caloric expenditure and, accordingly, durations as long as 40 to 60 minutes are recommended.

The prescription of exercise intensity for diabetics is similar to that for healthy adults (40 to 85% of functional capacity). However, non-insulin dependent diabetics should maintain an exercise intensity near the lower end of the functional capacity range (i.e., 40 to 60%) because their frequency and duration prescriptions are high. For most diabetic patients, the intensity may be prescribed by heart rate, however, for those with autonomic neuropathy and chronotropic insufficiency, heart rate prescription of intensity may be inappropriate. Therefore, exercise intensity may be best prescribed using RPE.

When beginning an exercise program, it may be important to monitor blood glucose before and after exercise to determine how exercise affects blood glucose levels in a given patient. Adjustments in carbohydrate intake and/or insulin may be needed as described above. In insulin-dependent diabetics there is a high risk of hypoglycemic reaction during or after (24 to 48 hours) exercise of higher intensity and longer duration. Patients with advanced retinopathy should not perform activities which cause excessive jarring or marked increases in blood pressure. Patients should have physician approval to resume exercise training following laser treatment.

OBESITY

Obesity may be defined as percent body fat that increases disease risk. The absolute percent body fat at which disease risk increases is controversial and this section will not address the issue of body composition standards for obesity. Rather, the focus is on methods for modifying the exercise prescription for those who are excessively fat.

As was discussed in Chapter 5, body fat is reduced when a chronic negative caloric balance exists. It is recommended that both an increase in caloric expenditure through exercise and a decrease in caloric intake be used to accomplish this goal. Exercise increases overall energy expenditure and also slows the rate of lean tissue loss that occurs when a person loses weight by dieting alone. This helps to maintain the resting metabolic rate and the rate of weight loss.

Obese subjects are usually sedentary and may have had a poor experience with exercise in the past. The exercise leader should interview the participant to determine past exercise history, potential scheduling difficulties, and the locations where exercise might be performed (e.g., sports club, home, street, school gym or track, etc.). This may increase adherence to an agreed upon exercise program.

The emphasis in exercise programming is on increasing caloric expenditure and minimizing the chances of muscle soreness, orthopedic injury, or other discomfort. Walking is often the exercise of choice, given that it is easy to schedule, the energy cost is predictable, and the stress on joints is minimal relative to other weight-bearing exercises. Alternative modes of exercise that reduce joint trauma include recumbent cycling, rowing, stair climbing and exercise in water. In the latter case, the energy cost of swimming per unit time is lower due to the greater buoyancy associated with the higher body fatness. However, walking or jogging through water that is waist or chest deep can result in a significant energy expenditure.

In contrast to the primary goal of achieving a cardiovascular training effect in most aerobic training programs, the primary goals for the obese subject are to establish a routine of exercise and achieve a reasonable energy expenditure during the activity. In the initial phase of the exercise program, the exercise intensity should be at or below the low end of the typical target heart rate range, with the duration of each session compensating to achieve an expenditure of 200 to 300 Kcal. The nature of low-intensity, low-impact exercise provides for the possibility of scheduling it on a daily basis. This approach results in a large number of calories expended per week.

On the basis of each person's response to the initial exercise program, in addition to their individual needs and goals, the exercise leader should adjust the intensity to bring the person into the target heart rate range. The higher intensity will allow for a shorter duration per session, or fewer sessions per week for the same weekly energy expenditure. In addition, the transition to higher intensity exercise will increase the number of opportunities to exercise with activities that naturally require a higher rate of energy expenditure. However, it must be added that for many, especially older subjects, a walking or other low-intensity exercise program may be all they desire, and movement toward a more intense program may be unwarranted. The exercise leader must match the needs and goals of the obese subject with the proper exercise program to achieve long-term weight management.

HYPERLIPIDEMIA

Hyperlipidemias contribute to atherosclerotic vascular diseases. High levels of low-density lipoprotein (LDL) and total cholesterol (TC) are known to accelerate the rate of atherogenesis, whereas high levels of high-density lipoprotein (HDL) are thought to protect against atherogenesis. The contributions of very low-density lipoprotein (VLDL) and triglycerides (TG) to atherogenesis are less well understood and are controversial. The lipoproteins are involved in metabolism of lipids and abnormalities in this system can cause hyperlipidemia and dyslipoproteinemia, of which there are several types. Some hyperlipidemias (types I, IIa, IIb, III) are the result of genetic abnormalities, while others are secondary to other co-existing conditions such as diabetes, obesity, alcohol abuse, oral contraceptive use, and pregnancy (types IV, V).

Treatment of hyperlipidemias include weight loss, dietary

reduction of fat intake, reduced cigarette and alcohol use, exercise and various pharmacological agents. Exercise and diet together may be effective in improving lipid profiles as well as reducing body fat. Exercise transiently reduces TG and VLDL, and chronic exercise has been shown to increase HDL (primarily the HDL_2 subfraction). The magnitude of change is usually 10 to 20% from diet and exercise therapy, so additional interventions may be necessary.

Exercise testing is required for these patients since hyperlipidemias contribute significantly to atherosclerosis. Conventional testing protocols are adequate for patients with hyperlipidemias. Exercise prescription should generally be focused on optimizing caloric expenditure. Therefore, durations up to 60 minutes and intensities near the lower end of the recommended range (40 to 60% $\dot{V}O_{2max}$) are suggested.

ARTHRITIS

Arthritis, a disease associated with inflammation of joint tissues, can result from two different disease processes: osteoarthritis or rheumatoid arthritis. Osteoarthritis (OA) is a progressive, irreversible degeneration of the articular surfaces of the joints. Rheumatoid arthritis (RA) is an autoimmune process that results in inflammation of the synovium—typically of distal joints. This immunologic disease often results in multisystemic involvement. Both result in painful inflammation of the joints, manifested by swelling and limited range of motion. RA patients experience periods of high arthritic activity interspersed with quiescent periods when little, if any, pain is experienced. In contrast, OA patients experience discomfort continuously. Patients are typically treated with analgesics and non-steroidal anti-inflammatory medications to reduce pain and inflammation. Glucocorticoids and other immunosuppressive agents are sometimes added for patients with RA who do not respond to initial therapy.

Exercise testing may be problematic in this patient group because their performance is primarily limited by joint pain instead of cardiovascular function. This often prevents the patients from achieving adequate myocardial stress and, therefore, reduces the diagnostic ability of the test. Non-weight bearing modes of exercise and/or arm ergometry may be useful because they avoid excessive joint stress and allow patients to attain a more reliable stress level.

Exercise prescription should be modified to include non-weight bearing activities in order to avoid excessive joint stress. Swimming may be the optimal exercise mode, although cycling and arm ergometry may be well tolerated. Activities which require quick movements are not advised. Specific strengthening and range of motion exercises should also be included to optimize joint stability and range of motion.

The exercise prescription must be flexible in terms of duration and intensity of exercise and will be dependent upon the disease activity and levels of pain experienced by the patient. Shorter duration with increased frequency (e.g., 15 minutes twice a day) may be indicated in some patients. During periods of high disease activity in RA patients, some minimal amount of physical activity should be performed to avoid the detrimental effects of bed rest and to maintain range of motion.

Exercise intensity should be at the level of pain tolerance of the individual on a given day. In patients with RA the intensity of exercise will be dramatically reduced during the inflammatory episodes. Actively inflamed joints indicate accelerated degeneration and may become worse with exercise. Patients are typically treated with analgesics and/or anti-inflammatory agents that may decrease the pain sensation experienced during exercise, possibly increasing the risk of tissue damage. Thus, during periods of severe inflammation in RA patients, caution must be taken to modify the mode of exercise to minimize any tissue damage.

END-STAGE RENAL DISEASE

Patients with end-stage renal disease (ESRD) have three treatment options: hemodialysis (most common), peritoneal dialysis and transplantation. The consequences of end-stage renal failure are multisystemic, especially in those treated with dialysis. Patients treated with hemodialysis must be connected to the artificial kidney machine for 3 to 4 hours, 3 times per week. They typically experience dramatic fluid shifts, electrolyte abnormalities, hypertension, and anemia. In the long term, many patients experience cardiovascular complications such as LVH and/or congestive heart failure from chronic volume and pressure overload. Virtually all risk factors for coronary artery disease tend to be present and there is a high prevalence of atherosclerosis in these patients. Other problems common in this patient group include: renal osteodystrophy, muscle weakness and cramping, lipid abnormalities, glucose intolerance, and depression. Many patients are also diabetic.

Most dialysis patients lead a sedentary existence and peak exercise tolerance is usually low (<5 METs). Exercise testing for diagnostic purposes may be of limited value due to significant peripheral limitation (muscle weakness) and a blunted heart rate response to exercise. Average peak heart rates have been reported to be only 70% of age-predicted levels. Thus, most patients are unable to achieve adequate myocardial stress to elicit diagnostic ECG changes. In addition, exercise ECGs may not be interpretable due to abnormalities caused by LVH and/or electrolyte imbalances. Exercise testing to evaluate functional capacity should incorporate a low level protocol with 1 MET (or less) increments between stages. Most patients exhibit hypertensive responses to exercise.

Exercise training can increase exercise tolerance and muscle strength in most patients and in some patients may increase hematocrit levels and improve blood pressure control and lipid profiles. Only patients who are on a stable regimen of dialysis, diet and medication should be considered for exercise training. The exercise prescription must be low level and walking, cycling and swimming are the most commonly recommended modes. Most patients should start with intervals of 3 to 4 minutes of exercise interspersed with rest periods. The exercise intervals should be gradually increased until 30 to 45 minutes of exercise can be performed. Initially a frequency of twice per day may be appropriate since the initial tolerable duration is so low. The intensity of exercise should be prescribed using RPE (12 to 13 on the 6 to 20 scale), since there is significant intra-individual variability in heart rate due to fluid status, medication schedule, and autonomic dysfunction.

Timing of exercise is another consideration in these patients. Hemodialysis patients may respond best to exercise on "non-dialysis" days. However, compliance and time factors often become problematic, making exercise training (cycling) during the hemodialysis treatment an appealing consideration. Such programming has been shown to be safe and it provides a medically monitored situation for exercise that may enhance exercise compliance. Exercise performed during the first 2 hours of the dialysis is usually well tolerated and does not interfere with the dialysis treatment.

Patients treated with peritoneal dialysis may choose to exercise during a dialysis exchange when their abdomen is completely or partially empty of fluid. Timing the exercise to an exchange may enhance participation by making it a part of the dialysis procedure. This timing may also result in the achievement of a higher training intensity because it is more comfortable for the patient and allows greater diaphragmatic movement. While swimming is not strictly contraindicated, there may be increased risk of infection if careful catheter care is not maintained.

Exercise training does not affect renal function, nor should it interfere with or affect the dialysis treatments. Most patients increase their functional capacity and muscle strength with exercise training. However, not all patients achieve expected health benefits (improved blood pressure control, lipids, etc.) from exercise training. This is especially likely in those who have multiple complicating pathologic conditions. It is therefore important to develop realistic expectations and to encourage individual patients to optimize their functional capacity. These goals and the recommendations for exercise prescription may change as therapy and technology improve. Two innovations that are currently being implemented are the administration of human recombinant erythropoietin for correction of the anemia and high-flux/high efficiency dialysis which shortens the hemodialysis treatment times.

ORGAN TRANSPLANTATION

Patients receiving organ transplants, such as liver and kidney, typically respond well to transplantation and are good candidates for exercise therapy. Recent advances in immunosuppression therapy have significantly improved graft and patient survival statistics. Rejection of the transplant and infection are primary concerns along with extreme deconditioning due to the sedentary lifestyle that typically exists prior to transplantation. Patients receiving renal transplants present with some or all of the complications of ESRD described previously. After transplantation many of these conditions are improved or reversed, however, patients are still at high risk for cardiovascular disease and most exhibit hypertension and hyperlipidemia. Patients chosen for liver transplantation typically have few coexisting medical problems (e.g., heart disease) that would complicate the procedure and recovery.

Exercise and other lifestyle interventions are critical following transplantation for several reasons. First, patients typically have been chronically ill for a prolonged period of time and often have required passive therapy (e.g., dialysis) for survival. Second, following transplantation patients must be re-oriented to healthy living and every effort should be made to prevent them from slipping back into a passive, "chronic disease" lifestyle. Third, immunosuppression medication includes the use of corticosteroids (specifically prednisone) which may cause proximal skeletal muscle wasting, redistribution of body fat to the torso area, increased appetite (with resulting significant weight gain), elevated lipids (primarily triglycerides and VLDL cholesterol) and, in some cases, aseptic necrosis of the hip or shoulder joints. Exercise training has been shown to counteract the loss of muscle strength and improve functional capacity. In conjunction with a low-fat/low-cholesterol diet and modification of eating habits to control food intake, exercise can help curb the severe weight gains typically experienced following transplantation.

Exercise therapy should begin as soon as possible after the surgery—often within 1 week when there are no complications. Initial therapy should consist of low-level strength training, using low resistances and high repetitions. Low-level aerobic exercise should be started early (often within the second postoperative week). Gradual progression of exercise to a duration of at least 30 to 45 minutes no less than 4 times per week should be the goal. Patients should be discharged with a plan for exercise that is considered an integral part of their medical therapy. Adherence may be promoted by including exercise on the medical log along with blood pressure, weight, etc.

As long as patients are not in rejection and have no other medical concerns that would contraindicate participation in physical activity, transplant patients may exercise in a manner similar to deconditioned healthy adults. Non-weight bearing activities are optimal to minimize joint stress. Jogging is typically not recommended due to the possibility of joint deterioration resulting from the prednisone. When exercise is appropriately prescribed and followed, these patients have the potential to progress and achieve normal levels of exercise tolerance. Patients who have adequate muscle strength and cardiorespiratory endurance should not be restricted in their sports participation (except for contact sports, which could damage the transplanted organ).

When working with immunosuppressed patients, utmost caution must be taken to protect patients from sources of infection. All personnel must practice standard infection control techniques. In addition, the following should be implemented:

1. All respiratory tubing and facemasks used for exercise testing should be sterilized prior to use (preferably in 12 to 18 hour Cidex-glutaraldehyde solution). Washing in soap or brief soaks in alcohol or bleach are not acceptable or adequate.
2. Exercise equipment, swimming pools, saunas, hot-tubs, and locker-rooms should be kept clean and should be checked daily to ensure compliance with (or superiority to) public health standards.
3. Exercise and testing personnel who may be carrying or suffering from a contagious process (colds, "flu," etc.) should avoid contact with patients during this time. In addition, they should not touch surfaces (i.e., sinks, door knobs, etc.) that patients may contact.

CANCER

Exercise therapy is becoming an accepted aspect of rehabilitation in patients with cancer. Regular exercise counteracts the detrimental effects of bed rest and provides psychological benefits. Also, exercise has been hypothesized to enhance immune function, and this would be especially beneficial in cancer patients.

Cancer is a host of diseases characterized by abnormal, unrestricted growth of cells that compress, invade, subvert and destroy adjacent body tissues. Malignant tumors are classified according to their tissue of origin, presence of lymph node invasion and possible metastases to other tissues. In addition to the effects of primary and secondary malignancies, the effects and side-effects of therapy must be considered in exercise testing, exercise prescription, and implementation of an exercise program. Cancer treatments include surgery, radiotherapy, chemotherapy, and immunotherapy and these are often associated with cytotoxicity, immunologic suppression, prolonged bleeding, and other side-effects such as fatigue. Malignancy-related crises such as pathological bone fractures, chemotherapy-induced cardiac or pulmonary damage, anemia, low platelet count, tumor-host competition for nutrients, dehydration, electrolyte imbalances, and opportunistic infections are problems that must be constantly evaluated with respect to exercise programming. Exercise therapy must be a part of a coordinated medical therapy and the physician who is primarily responsible for the patient's care must be involved in the decision to initiate exercise training.

Exercise tolerance may be affected by any number of factors resulting from the disease and/or treatment. It has been reported that peak exercise capacity is often in the range of 3 to 5 METs. Cardiopulmonary testing may be important to determine the limitations of that system before starting exercise. Patients with actual or potential metastases to the bone (most notably spine, pelvis, femur, and ribs) should be tested using cycle ergometers. Non-weight bearing exercises may also be appropriate for exercise training.

The exercise prescription for intensity should be at the lower end of the heart rate reserve (40 to 65%) and adjusted as tolerated by the patient. Interval/intermittent exercise training on a cycle ergometer at an intensity of 60 to 75% of peak heart rate has been tolerated in ambulatory patients and has been successful in producing significant changes in functional capacity.

Exercise frequency is determined by the clinical status of the patient. In these patients many factors can be encountered that indicate modification of the exercise prescription (e.g., decrease intensity) or deferring exercise to another time or day. Such conditions include: presence of intravenous devices required for chemotherapy which may be dislodged during activity and stretching; fatigue, nausea, and malaise following administration of medication or radiation therapy; muscle weakness, dehydration, and any pain or cramping. Toxicity from medical treatments may result in low blood counts (platelets <50,000; white blood cells <3000), fever (>100°F), low hemoglobin levels (<10 g/dl), muscle weakness, numbness in the extremities, extreme fatigue and may preclude exercise training.

Dynamic lifting exercise to maintain or enhance muscle strength is important and should be performed on machines rather than with free weights to avoid any potential for bruising or bone fractures and because patients may experience neuromuscular symptoms and problems with balance. Low-resistance, high repetition workouts are recommended. Patients with low platelet counts should avoid resistance training 36 hours prior to venipuncture for enzyme studies since there is a concern about the effect of resistance training on enzymes that may be used in following the clinical course of the patients.

SPECIAL CONDITIONS WITHIN THE NORMAL POPULATION

The following sections address recommended procedures for exercise prescription in three nondiseased special populations. These three groups are children, the elderly and pregnant women. For each of these groups unique physiologic and behavioral characteristics require that special considerations be applied in designing exercise programs.

PREGNANCY

Pregnant women represent a unique exercising group because of the possible competition between exercising maternal muscle and the fetus for blood flow, oxygen delivery, glucose availability, and heat dissipation. Also, metabolic and cardiorespiratory adaptations to pregnancy may alter the responses to acute exercise and the adaptations that result from exercise training. Benefits that are reasonable to expect from a properly designed prenatal exercise program include: improved aerobic and muscular fitness, facilitation of labor and recovery from labor, enhanced maternal psychological well-being, and establishment of permanent healthy lifestyle habits.

Exercise responses, and therefore the exercise prescription, may change during the course of the pregnancy. Some experts have expressed concern that during the first trimester exercise-induced hyperthermia may affect the closure of the neural tube. Also, the possibility of competing maternal and fetal physiological needs is greatest during exercise in the third trimester. Thus, it is probably not advisable for pregnant women to begin a NEW strenuous exercise program during the first or third trimesters. However, existing scientific studies generally support the concept that gradual increases in physical activity are appropriate during the second trimester when the discomforts and possible risks of exercise are low. Intensity and duration of an ongoing exercise program should not be increased during the third trimester and should be decreased if there are signs of exertional intolerance and chronic fatigue.

Although some pregnant women have undergone maximal exercise testing, this is not recommended in nonclinical settings. Women who are appropriately screened prior to initiating exercise and who are educated regarding signs and/or symptoms for discontinuing exercise typically do not experience problems. Contraindications for exercise during pregnancy have been established by the American College of Obstetrics and Gynecology (ACOG) and are listed in Table 7–1.

The best modes of exercise during pregnancy are walking and non-weight bearing activities such as stationary cycling or exercise in water. For already exercising women, athletic training for competition should be discontinued. As pregnancy progresses, the center of gravity shifts and may alter balance for safe sports participation. Performance of flexibility exercises has been discouraged due to the looseness of joints, however, stretching to relieve muscle soreness for postural imbalance may be beneficial. LaMaze exercise can complement aerobic training and be helpful in the birthing process. The use of weight training for muscular conditioning during pregnancy is controversial. Any exercise that positions the individual in the supine posture during later gestation should be avoided because of a risk of postural hypotension. The pregnant uterus may compress the descending aorta and inferior vena cava resulting in decreased cardiac output and decreased blood flow to the fetus.

Since a major goal of exercise training during pregnancy is

Table 7–1. Contraindications for Exercise During Pregnancy*

Absolute Contraindications	*Relative Contraindications*
Heart disease	High blood pressure
Ruptured membranes	Anemia or other blood disorders
Premature labor	Thyroid disease
Multiple gestation	Diabetes
Bleeding	Palpitations or irregular heart rhythms
Placenta previa	Breech presentation in the last trimester
Incompetent cervix	Excessive obesity
History of 3 or more spontaneous abortions or miscarriages	Extreme underweight
	History of precipitous labor
	History of intrauterine growth retardation
	History of bleeding during pregnancy
	Extremely sedentary lifestyle

*American College of Obstetricians and Gynecologists: *Exercise During Pregnancy and Postnatal Period (ACOG) Home Exercise Programs.* Washington DC: ACOG, 1985.

to maintain physical work capacity, the appropriate frequency of exercise is 3 to 5 times per week. Durations of 15 to 30 minutes are usually well tolerated. It is important to avoid exposing the fetus to prolonged hypoxic or thermal stresses, therefore longer duration exercise is not recommended.

Prescription of exercise intensity is complicated during pregnancy since resting heart rate is increased throughout pregnancy and maximal heart rate may be reduced in later gestation. Thus, use of conventional heart rate target zones to prescribe exercise intensity is less reliable than in non-pregnant subjects. Available data suggest that perception of exertion remains stable regardless of pregnancy status and therefore, use of RPE scales is highly recommended. A target intensity of approximately 12 to 14 on the 6 to 20 point Borg scale is appropriate for most pregnant women. An additional method of preventing over-exertion is to employ the "talk test." The talk test indicates that the intensity is excessive if an individual cannot carry on a verbal conversation during exercise.

The following precautions for the exercising pregnant woman should be strictly applied. A transition from weight bearing to non-weight bearing activity is recommended as body weight increases. High ambient temperatures and humidities should be avoided during exercise due to problems in thermoregulation during pregnancy. Supine exercise after the fourth month has been identified as problematic, although some individuals may tolerate supine exercise without experiencing problems. Exercise should be discontinued and a physician consulted when any of the symptoms listed in Table 7–2 are present.

After delivery, exercise can be resumed 8 weeks postpartum or as advised by the obstetrician. Guidelines for mode, fre-

Table 7–2. Signs and Symptoms for Discontinuing Exercise During Pregnancy*

Pain or bleeding
Dizziness or faintness
Pubic pain
Palpitations
Back pain
Rapid heart rates
Shortness of breath
Difficulty in walking

*American College of Obstetricians and Gynecologists: *Exercise During Pregnancy and Postnatal Period (ACOG) Home Exercise Programs.* Washington DC: ACOG, 1985.

quency and duration of exercise as presented in Chapter 5 are appropriate.

CHILDREN

Regular, vigorous exercise is to be encouraged in children and the American College of Sports Medicine has issued an Opinion Statement on this topic.[2] However, because youngsters are anatomically, physiologically, and psychologically immature, certain special precautions should be applied when designing exercise programs for them. A primary physiologic concern in exercising children is their ability to adapt to thermal stress. Thermoregulation in children during heat exposure is less efficient due to a higher threshold for sweating and lower output of heat-activated sweat glands. Although children have a lower body mass to surface area ratio, the efficiency of heat loss through conduction, radiation, and convection may be low due to lower skin blood flow rates in children. Thus, children appear to be more prone than adults to heat injury. Also, the low body mass to surface area in children results in accelerated heat loss during exposure to cold, which increases their risk of hypothermia.

Children are physiologically adaptive to endurance exercise training. However, concern has been expressed that children may experience a higher incidence of overuse injuries or damage the epiphyseal growth plates if the quantity of endurance exercise is excessive. Although there are no conclusive studies that address these concerns, persons who design training programs for children should be encouraged to: (1) increase the quantity of exercise gradually; (2) assure adequate muscular strength and flexibility; (3) assure proper body mechanics; (4) assure the use of proper footwear and appropriate running surfaces; and (5) take appropriate precautions in high temperature environments, such as limiting strenuous prolonged exercise, providing adequate hydration and encouraging light clothing.

Evidence suggests that children can participate safely in properly designed progressive strength training programs with close adult supervision. Children can significantly increase strength via such programs, and percentage improvements in performance are comparable to those of adults.

THE ELDERLY

Goals for physical activity in this population include maintenance of functional capacity for independent living, reduction in the risk of cardiovascular disease, retardation of the progression of chronic diseases, promotion of psychological well-being and provision of opportunities for social interaction. Physiological changes occurring with age are variable and some that may alter the exercise prescription include reductions in maximal aerobic power, cardiovascular reserve (primarily due to lower maximal heart rate), elasticity of the peripheral vasculature, heat tolerance, muscular strength, elasticity of connective tissue, and musculoskeletal flexibility. Additionally, there is a higher prevalence of symptomatic and asymptomatic CAD and other chronic diseases such as hypertension, diabetes mellitus, degenerative bone and joint diseases, and malnutrition. Thus, individualization of the exercise prescription is essential and should be based on the health status and individual goals of the participant.

Assessment of physical fitness is difficult in the elderly since standard test batteries and norms for evaluation are not readily available for this population. Since there is a high prevalence of cardiovascular disease and risk factors for CAD in the elderly, exercise testing is typically recommended prior to beginning a strenuous exercise program (see Chapter 1). The exercise prescription should be developed from the results of this test and individualized according to the specific needs of the participant (see Chapter 5). Walking, chair and floor exercises, and modified strength/flexibility calisthenics are well-tolerated by most elderly individuals. Water exercise, swimming or cycling may be more appropriate for those with bone/joint problems.

REFERENCES

1. American College of Obstetricians and Gynecologists: *Exercise During Pregnancy and Postnatal Period (ACOG) Home Exercise Programs.* Washington D.C.: ACOG, 1985.
2. American College of Sports Medicine: Opinion statement on physical fitness in children and youth. *Med Sci Sports Exerc 20*:422–423, 1988.
3. Artal R and Wiswell RA (eds.): *Exercise in Pregnancy.* Baltimore: Williams & Wilkins, 1986.
4. Cox NJ, VanHarwaarden CL, Fogering H and Binkhorst RA: Exercise and training in patients with chronic obstructive lung disease. *Sports Med 6*:180–192, 1988.
5. Fletcher GF (ed): *The Use of Exercise in the Practice of Medicine.* Mt Kisco, NY: Futura Publishing Co, 1982.
6. Franklin B (ed): *Exerise in Modern Medicine.* Baltimore: Williams & Wilkins, 1988.
7. Gisolfi CV and Lamb DR (eds): *Perspectives in Exercise Science and Sports*

Medicine Vol 2: Youth, Exercise and Sports. Indianapolis: Benchmark Press, 1989.

8. Goldberg AP, Geltman EM, Hagberg JM, Gavin JR, Delmez JM, Carney RM, Naumowicz A, Oldfield MH and Harter HR: The therapeutic effects of exercise training for hemodialysis patients. *Kidney Int 24*(suppl 16):S303–S309, 1983.
9. Gorski J: Exercise during pregnancy: maternal and fetal responses. A brief review. *Med Sci Sports Exerc 17*:407–416, 1985.
10. Horber FF, Scheidegger JR, Grunig BE and Frey FJ: Evidence that prednisone-induced myopathy is reversed by physical training. *J Clin Endocrinol Metab 61*:83–88, 1985.
11. Kremmer FW and Berger M: Exercise and diabetes mellitus: Physical activity as a part of daily life and its role in the treatment of diabetic patients. *Int J Sports Med 4*:77–88, 1983.
12. MacVicar MG, Winningham ML and Nickel JL: Effects of aerobic interval training in cancer patients' functional capacity. *Nurs Res 38*:348–351, 1989.
13. Micheli LJ: Pediatric and adolescent sports injuries. *Exerc Sport Sci Rev 14*:349–351, 1986.
14. Miller TD, Squires RW, Gau GT, Frohnert PR and Sterioff S: Graded exercise testing and training after renal transplantation. A preliminary study. *Mayo Clin Proc 62*:773–777, 1987.
15. Painter PL, Nelson-Worel JN, Hill MM, Thornbery DR, Shelp WR, Harrington AR and Weinstein AB: Effects of exercise training during hemodialysis. *Nephron 43*:87–92, 1986.
16. Painter PL: Exercise in end-stage renal disease. *Exerc Sport Sci Rev 16*:305–339, 1988.
17. Pate RR and Ward DS: Endurance exercise trainability in children and youth. In *Advances in Sports Medicine and Fitness,* Vol. 3. Edited by WA Grana, JA Lombardo, BJ Sharkey and JA Stone. Chicago: Year Book Medical Publishers, Inc., 1990.
18. Richter EA and Ruderman NB: Diabetes and exercise. *Am J Med 70*:201–209, 1981.
19. Roman O, Camuzzi AL, Villalon E and Klenner C: Physical training program in arterial hypertension: A long-term prospective follow-up. *Cardiology 67*:230–243, 1981.
20. Ruttenberg HD, Moller JH, Strang WB, Fisher AG and Adams TD: Recommended guidelines for graded exercise testing and exercise prescription for children with heart disease. *J Cardiac Rehabil 4*:10–16, 1984.
21. Schulman SP and Gerstenblith G: Guidelines for the exercise training of elderly healthy individuals and elderly patients with cardiac disease. *J Cardiopul Rehabil 9*:40–45, 1989.
22. Seales D and Hagberg J: The effect of exercise training on human hypertension: A review. *Med Sci Sports Exerc 16*:207–215, 1984.
23. Skinner JS (ed): *Exercise Testing and Exercise Prescription for Special Cases. Theoretical Basis and Clinical Application.* Philadelphia: Lea & Febiger, 1987.
24. Stamford B: Exercise and the elderly. *Exerc Sport Sci Rev 16*:341–379, 1988.
25. Symposium: Exercise in the treatment of obesity. *Med Sci Sports Exerc 18*:1–30, 1986.

26. Thompson JK, Jarvie GJ, Lahey BB and Cureton KJ: Exercise and obesity: Etiology, physiology and intervention. *Psychol Bull 91*:55–79, 1982.
27. Vistug A, Schneider SH and Ruderman NB: Exercise and type I diabetes mellitus. *Exerc Sport Sci Rev 16*:285–304, 1988.
28. Winningham ML: Cancer and exercise. In *Exercise as Medical Therapy: Physiologic Principles and Clinical Considerations.* Edited by L Goldberg and DL Elliot. Philadelphia: FA Davis, 1990.
29. Wolfe LA, Ohtake PJ, Mottola MF and McGrath MJ: Physiological interactions between pregnancy and aerobic exercise. *Exerc Sport Sci Rev 17*:295–351, 1989.

CHAPTER 8

Methods for Changing Health Behaviors

EXERCISE AND THE HEALTHY LIFESTYLE

By current standards, a person is not considered truly healthy unless he or she practices a lifestyle that reduces the risks of the major chronic diseases. Regular exercise is an important part of "behavioral health," but many participants in exercise programs are also interested in improving their dietary and smoking habits, achieving or maintaining ideal weight, or managing stress effectively. Whether the exercise program serves primarily healthy individuals or medical patients, exercise is likely to be just one of the health behaviors that program participants are attempting to change. Exercise program personnel should be aware of and support efforts to change all of these health behaviors.

Making lifestyle changes of any kind is difficult, and exercise may be more difficult to change than some other behaviors. Many beginning exercise program staff, being immersed in exercise science and surrounded every day by committed exercisers, expect that program participants will become committed exercisers once they learn the many benefits of exercise. These staff members may then become disillusioned and frustrated when attendance to exercise sessions is sporadic and many participants drop out of the program. The research on exercise adherence has revealed that 50% of participants drop out within 1 year. Knowledge about the benefits of exercise and motivation do not predict behavior well. Simply cajoling participants and giving pep talks is unlikely to be effective. There are some specific steps that exercise program staff can take that will help participants exercise regularly. In the next section some of these techniques are briefly described.

INITIATING AND MAINTAINING EXERCISE BEHAVIOR: APPLICATION OF BEHAVIORAL PRINCIPLES

The methods of behavior change presented here are based upon literally thousands of human and animal studies in behavior modification and behavior therapy. These specific techniques are effective in changing many kinds of behaviors, but their use does not guarantee success. The techniques presented here should be integrated into the exercise program in a way that is appropriate to the population, the setting, and the skill level of the staff, based on professional judgment. An effective program would selectively incorporate several of these techniques into a coherent multicomponent program, but it is not necessary to use all of them. Because all exercise program staff are attempting to change behavior, course work or directed readings in scientifically validated approaches to behavior change are strongly recommended. The techniques are only introduced in this chapter, so additional readings, relevant training, or consultation from an expert in behavior change will be needed. The *Resource Manual for Guidelines for Exercise Testing and Prescription* contains several chapters that provide additional information about principles of health behavior change,[17] group exercise leadership,[16] and improving exercise adherence.[11] The chapter by Knapp[12] contains a great deal of information on behavior change techniques as does Williams and Long.[19] For an in-depth, yet practical, approach to behavior change methods, Kanfer and Goldstein[10] is an excellent volume.

Following the organization of Martin and Dubbert,[13] techniques are grouped according to whether they are most applicable to promoting initiation or maintenance of exercise.

INITIATION OF EXERCISE

Preparation. For those beginning an exercise program, it is important to have reasonable expectations. The exercise leader should ask new participants what they expect to gain by exercise and in what period of time. Overly pessimistic (e.g., "no pain, no gain") and overly optimistic (e.g., "I want the runner's high") expectations should be corrected. Participants should be told what benefits they can reasonably expect and what amount of exercise is needed to achieve those benefits.

In an introductory interview or meeting it is helpful to have the new participant make a firm commitment to stay with the program for a specified length of time (e.g., 3 to 6 months) to give the program a fair chance to produce some benefits. This commitment can be verbal, but it is more effective to have a written contract (see below).

Shaping. The behavioral principle of shaping is analogous to the physiological principle of progression. This principle recognizes that behavior is best changed gradually. Begin the exercise program at a volume (intensity, frequency, duration) that is comfortable for the individual, and increase the volume slowly until the prescribed level is reached. It is preferable to begin at a volume that is too low rather than too high. Starting at a level that is too advanced may be aversive to someone who is unfamiliar with exercise. Starting at a low level and increasing the volume will enhance participants' self-confidence and motivation to continue.

Goal-setting. The leader and the participant should jointly set exercise goals that will ensure a gradual progression. It is important that the goals be individualized and based upon the participant's physiological capacity and perceived ability to achieve the goals. Goals can be set for both supervised and unsupervised exercise, if appropriate. Short-term goals that cover 1 or 2 weeks are more effective than longer term goals. Goals should be specific and state the dates, times, and places of the planned exercise sessions. Goals should be flexible, such that if one session is missed, it can be made up on another day. At the end of each goal period, performance should be evaluated. Successes and problems in meeting the goal should be discussed, and new goals should be set. It is essential to review performance and give feedback to the participant about his or her progress.

Reinforcement. Reinforcement (also known as "rewards") is the most effective method for changing behavior. In fact, a reinforcer is defined as anything that is presented during or after the behavior that increases the probability of the occurrence of that behavior. Participants should have a role in suggesting what reinforcers would work for them. What is a good reinforcer for one person may not be effective for another person. However, numerous rewards systems should be built into the program. One of the most effective rewards may be praise from program staff during and just after the exercise session. Staff should provide praise that is specific to each individual. The exercise itself should be as reinforcing as possible so that the participant enjoys the type and intensity of the workout. Lotteries and point systems that allow the participants to earn tangible reinforcers have been effective in some studies. Participants can deposit money at the beginning of the program that is returned at intervals, based upon attendance. Simple symbolic rewards can also be effective, such as making public charts of attendance, miles covered, etc. Certificates, patches, and buttons can also be used as reinforcers at low cost. Periodic fitness testing with feedback and interpretation of results can be an effective reinforcer.

Stimulus Control. Environmental cues or stimuli in the home, work place, or program setting may remind or encourage participants to become regular in their exercise habits. Many stimulus control strategies can be devised: write exercise time in appointment books, set watch alarms for exercise time, put up written reminders, lay out exercise clothes the night before, plan to meet friends for exercise, go to the exercise facility even when you do not feel like exercising, and talk every day with friends who exercise. Having a routine time and place for exercise, either with the group or independently, establishes powerful stimulus control. Phoning frequently absent participants the day before the scheduled session may be an effective cue to attendance.

Contracting. A behavioral contract specifies the relationship between the exercise behavior and the reinforcement. The contract is used for formalizing a commitment to exercise. The participant can negotiate a contract with program staff, the physicians, the spouse, or a friend. The participant agrees to perform a given level of exercise for a specified amount of time, and the other person agrees to reinforce that behavior in a specified manner. The reinforcement may be praise, a desired tangible item (e.g., a sweat suit) or a privilege (e.g., going to a concert). Contracts not only provide a written record of the entire exercise plan, but they are an excellent vehicle for involving significant others in the exercise program. Signing the contract formalizes the agreement and makes it more important. The contract ties together many of the behavioral methods and insures that the plans are specific enough to write down. Contracts should specify short-term goals and focus on *positive* consequences for achievement of the goal. At the end of the contract period, they can be renegotiated and renewed.

Cognitive Strategies. A number of approaches to changing cognitions or thoughts related to exercise have been shown to be effective. Having participants systematically consider the advantages and disadvantages of exercise (i.e., the "balance sheet" decision method) can have at least a short-term effect on participation.[18] Participants who select their own flexible goals based on exercise time, rather than distance covered, will probably attend better than those participants whose goals are rigidly dictated by exercise leaders. While athletes are often taught to focus attention on their bodily sensations, this may be counterproductive for beginners. Noncompetitive exercisers usually find it more appealing to concentrate on the external environment (e.g., "smell the roses") so they are distracted from any discomfort associated with the exercise.

MAINTENANCE OF EXERCISE

Generalization Training. In programs where the participant is not expected to exercise under supervision indefinitely, specific steps need to be taken to "generalize" the exercise habit from the program setting to the home setting. This process can start early in the program by helping participants set up home exercise programs to supplement supervised exercise. In rehabilitation programs, generalization would not begin until it was clinically indicated. Generalization training is even needed in home programs, because many people simply stop exercising when they are away from home.

In supervised programs, home exercise sessions should be encouraged early, using the same exercise stimulus in both settings. Participants should record relevant data such as where, when, with whom, exercise type, intensity (including exercise heart rate), enjoyment, and problems. Discussion and resolution of problems early in the process can enhance long-term success of the home program.

Social Support. Social support is an extremely powerful influence on exercise behavior both in the early phases and the maintenance phase. The assistance of spouse, family members, friends, and co-workers should be elicited from the beginning. Leaders can promote the formation of pairs of "buddies," and buddies should contact one another on days between sessions to discuss progress and problems with exercise. Participants can ask friends and relatives to encourage them to exercise and to praise them for exercising. Finding a compatible exercise partner for a home or supervised program means the difference between success and failure for many people. Behavioral contracts should be encouraged between spouses or others in the participant's natural environment.

Self-Management. External reinforcement is useful for establishing the behavior initially, but self-management is much more effective for long-term maintenance. While social support from friends and relatives will continue to be reinforcing, participants should practice self-reinforcement by focusing on increased feelings of self-esteem, enjoyment from the stimulation of exercise itself, and anticipated health benefits. Participants can be taught to monitor and graph their own exercise behavior and to develop their own contracts and self-reinforcement strategies. The participants gradually learn how to be their own behavior therapists, and they can use these methods to maintain their exercise well after the program has ended.

Relapse Prevention Training. Despite the skillful application of the best available behavior change methods, most participants will eventually, at least briefly, lapse to a sedentary pattern. The goal of the leader is to prepare participants for the occurrence of such lapses and ways of coping with them so that a complete relapse is avoided. By laying the groundwork with social support and training in self-management and other skills, the frequency and length of relapses may be reduced. However, the way participants deal with relapses when they occur is important. The likelihood of relapses should be discussed, because relapses will not seem so disastrous if they are predicted ahead of time. There is little point in worrying about whether such frank discussion will produce relapses since almost everyone relapses at some time. Participants are taught to anticipate situations that would likely produce a relapse. For example, illness, travel, live-in visitors, overwork, bad weather, and emotional distress are commonly cited. Participants can prepare to avoid relapsing in some of these situations, and some high-risk situations can be avoided altogether. When relapses occur, it is critical for participants to view them not as failures but as challenges. As soon after the relapse as possible, it is important to apply self-management strategies to begin the exercise program again. Specifically, goals should be set, social support should be sought, and self-reinforcement should be reinstituted on a temporary basis.

SPECIAL POPULATIONS

Research on exercise determinants has shown that some types of people are more likely to drop out of exercise than others.[8]

The obese, blue collar workers, the elderly, smokers, and depressed individuals appear particularly prone to drop out. The exercise leader can, therefore, consider these types of individuals as "high risk," although the risk for dropout in all subgroups is high. Nevertheless, these special populations can be provided with additional support. Be alert for signs of discomfort while exercising or dissatisfaction with the program. Ask periodically how they are enjoying the exercise and if they are having any problems. Identifying counter-productive attitudes and beliefs (e.g., "I should be losing weight faster") can be useful. More frequent praise, individual attention, and assistance with self-management is indicated.

Poor attendance should be identified early in the program through attendance logs or other methods. In an individual conversation, the exercise leader should assess the cause of missed sessions and establish a plan for improving attendance. Assignment of regular participants to work with low-attendance participants harnesses powerful peer support and can be an effective technique. While individual attention is often helpful in improving attendance, it can become so time-consuming that it interferes with the total program. As a last resort, a contract may be developed that states if attendance falls below an agreed-upon level, the participant will be terminated from the program.

Since emotional problems, especially depression, are common, exercise leaders will encounter from time to time individuals in need of psychological counseling. If a participant appears to be particularly sad, prone to crying, or complains of sleep or appetite problems, you may want to gently ask them if they are feeling "under stress," "down," or "blue." If they indicate they are having emotional problems, ask if they would like help in getting counseling from a local mental health clinic or professional. Then assist them in calling to make an appointment with an appropriate professional.

OTHER TARGETS FOR HEALTH BEHAVIOR CHANGE

Exercise program personnel are often asked questions about other aspects of health lifestyles. While the exercise leader should not be expected to be an expert in all these areas, it is appropriate for him or her to serve as a resource person and to direct the participant to accurate information. Upon intake, it may be worthwhile to routinely assess other behaviors such as smoking status, body composition, diet (including consumption of high-fat foods), and perceived mood or level of stress. Based on initial screening tests participants could be counseled regarding the need for further assessment or behavior change. A short list of qualified local professionals and services related to each of these areas should be developed. The interested participants can be referred to people with whom the program develops a relationship over time.

SMOKING

Smoking is the largest preventable cause of death, so every health professional has an obligation to strongly urge smokers to quit. The exercise program staff can play an important role in helping smokers quit. Particularly after establishing rapport with clients and in the context of showing concern, program staff should ask if they want to quit and encourage them to do so. The following considerations may be useful in providing assistance.

1. Provide information on the dangers of smoking and the benefits of quitting. The connections between smoking and the symptoms they are having, medical findings, or other relevant concerns should be detailed. Emphasize that quitting smoking is probably the single most important action they can take to improve their health
2. Determine the participant's willingness to quit
3. Evaluate past failures and develop new strategies
4. Request a quit date and develop a specific cessation plan
5. Provide a list of programs (detailed by phone number, address, method, and cost) and have available handouts (for instance the National Cancer Institute's or American Lung Association's self-help smoking cessation materials)
6. Follow up and provide encouragement and support
7. Prepare for relapse

For participants who simply refuse to quit at this time, ask them if you can inquire about quitting in the future, and do so. Individuals not willing to quit at one time may change their mind later on and will benefit from a kind but firm continued reminder of the importance of stopping. Additional information on smoking cessation can be found in the ACSM Resource Manual.[9]

When there is some interest in quitting, then smokers should be provided with either some materials to help them quit on their own or a referral to one or more high-quality smoking cessation clinics.

Self-help materials based on empirical research are available at low cost from:

"Quit for Good" Kit
Office of Cancer Communications
National Cancer Institute
Bldg. 31, Room 10A18
Bethesda, MD 20205

Stanford Health Promotion
Resource Center
1000 Welch Road
Palo Alto, CA 94304-1885
415-723-1000

Local chapters of the American Lung Association and the American Cancer Society usually either sponsor smoking cessation services or compile lists of local programs. National offices can supply the phone number of local chapters.

American Lung Association
1740 Broadway
New York, NY 10019
212-315-8700

American Cancer Society
1599 Clifton Road
Atlanta, GA 30329
404-320-3333

OVERWEIGHT

Available evidence indicates that the prevalence of moderate to severe obesity is high. While a few people are overweight because of hormonal or other physical disorders, the majority who are excessively fat exercise too little relative to caloric intake. Permanent weight loss can occur by decreasing food consumption and by increasing energy expended through physical activity. Many studies have shown that the adoption of a physical activity program is the best predictor of long-term weight loss and its subsequent maintenance. Many self-help, therapist-aided, or group programs which teach new eating habits and encourage physical activity are available and lead to a realistic and safe rate of weight loss of approximately 1 kg per week.

A participant can be helped with a weight loss program in several ways.

1. Emphasize the importance of gradual weight loss based on changes in the diet (decreased caloric intake) and increased physical activity. There are many specific behavioral recommendations for weight reduction. For example: keep a food diary; eat only fruit for snacks; reduce fried

foods; eat meatless meals; chew food thoroughly; put down fork between bites; and use a small plate
2. Review the participant's past successes and failures with weight loss
3. Establish realistic short and long-term goals. Avoid fad diets or fasts
4. Provide appropriate written support and instructional materials
5. Prepare the client for relapses (for instance, do not become discouraged after a high calorie binge) or plateaus of weight loss (more exercise, or fewer calories might be indicated)
6. Continue to monitor the person's progress and provide support and encouragement

Since change in body composition should be a gradual process, with occasional lack of progress likely to occur, the program staff should assume a patient, nonjudgmental attitude. Additional information on weight loss can be found in the ACSM Resource Manual.[3]

Many weight loss books can be found in any bookstore. Many of these promote unproven or even dangerous methods, so the exercise leader should investigate the bookstores periodically and be able to recommend books that are based on current research. There is little evidence that people are able to lose weight simply with the aid of a book, so obese participants should be counseled to join a reputable program. Credible programs employ procedures that are consistent with the guidelines described above. Such programs are available in most communities.

DIET

The typical American diet is high in calories, fat (particularly saturated fat), cholesterol, and sodium, and it is low in fiber. This dietary pattern contributes to a number of chronic diseases.

The chief goals of dietary change are often to:
1. Reduce or maintain body weight
2. Reduce elevated plasma total and LDL-cholesterol
3. Reduce blood pressure

These goals are achieved through appropriate changes in calories, saturated fat, cholesterol, and salt intake as suggested by the Senate Select Committee's Dietary Goals for the Nation.

Permanent adoption of an eating style that helps a person lose weight, lower cholesterol, and/or reduce sodium intake, usually requires a slow but persistent change in eating habits. The following steps may be useful:

1. Provide information to the participant as to the need for change and the advantages of doing so
2. Establish a baseline of the participant's current dietary intake. Computerized analysis of 24-hour dietary intake, 4 to 7 day food diaries, or standardized diet history can be used for this purpose
3. Establish concrete short-term goals related to menu planning, shopping, snacking, eating out, and cooking methods. Specific foods or dietary practices should be targeted. The participant should be asked to make commitments to achieving these goals, and behavioral contracts can be helpful in formalizing the goals and commitment.
4. Provide appropriate nutrition, food preparation, and other relevant materials
5. Continue to follow the participant's progress in reaching the short-term goals. As short-term goals are reached, new goals should be established until the long-term dietary changes are reached

A well-trained exercise leader may be able to provide assistance for achieving the above steps, but consultation with a dietitian is also important. Additional information on nutrition can be found in the ACSM Resource Manual.[4]

For a healthy person there are a number of books that can be used as a guide to dietary change and some of these are included in the reference list.[2,5,6] Additional materials are available from the Stanford Health Promotion Resource Center (see address above).

For patients under treatment or others with specialized needs, the best source of information and assistance is a registered dietitian (R.D.). They are listed in the yellow pages.

STRESS MANAGEMENT

"Stress" is a popular term that is used to refer to everything from daily annoyances to major emotional disorders. Exercise can help alleviate feelings of distress and mild depression, so it is a proper coping technique for minor emotional problems. In addition, there are specific stress management methods that have been shown to reduce psychological and physiological symptoms of stress.

Stress management techniques aimed at altering physiological variables (like blood pressure or heart rate), inducing a general state of relaxation and well-being, changing behavior patterns, enhancing coping mechanisms, or combinations of these techniques are becoming increasingly popular. Stress management programs include avoidance techniques where the participant avoids the stressful situation, adjustment/adaptation techniques where the participant copes more appropriately with the stressor, or alteration techniques like relaxation and biofeedback which normalize physiological reactions to stress. The specific stress management techniques to be used remain controversial. Most people can easily learn a relaxation procedure, but other stress management techniques may require more intensive instruction by a psychotherapist. Additional information on stress management can be found in the ACSM Resource Manual.[15]

For those who want to learn safe and effective methods of relaxing, there are many books and cassette tapes.[1] Group stress management programs are commonly offered by health promotion programs, hospitals, and private practitioners. Reputable local programs should be identified.

Participants with emotional disorders should be referred to a licensed psychiatrist, psychologist, or social worker. A few individual practitioners should be identified and kept on hand for referrals.

REFERENCES

1. Benson H: *The Relaxation Response.* New York: Aron, 1975.
2. Brody JE: *Jane Brody's Nutrition Book: A Lifetime Guide to Good Eating for Better Health and Weight Control.* New York: Horton, 1981.
3. Brownell KD: Weight management and body composition. In *Resource Manual for Guidelines for Exercise Testing and Prescription.* Edited by American College of Sports Medicine. Philadelphia: Lea & Febiger, 1988.
4. Brownell KD and Steen SN: Nutrition. In *Resource Manual for Guidelines for Exercise Testing and Prescription.* Edited by American College of Sports Medicine. Philadelphia: Lea & Febiger, 1988.
5. Cooper KH: *Controlling Cholesterol.* New York: Bantam, 1988.
6. Connor SJ and Connor WE: *The New American Diet.* New York: Simon & Schuster, 1986.
7. Dishman RK (Ed): *Exercise Adherence: Its Impact on Public Health.* Champaign, IL: Human Kinetics, 1988.
8. Dishman RK, Sallis JF and Orenstein DM: The determinants of physical activity and exercise. *Public Health Rep 100*:158–172, 1985.

9. Gottlieb AN and Sachs DPL: Smoking cessation. In *Resource Manual for Guidelines for Exercise Testing and Prescription.* Edited by American College of Sports Medicine. Philadelphia: Lea & Febiger, 1988.
10. Kanfer FH and Goldstein AP (Eds): *Helping People Change: A Textbook of Methods,* 3rd Ed. New York: Pergamon, 1988.
11. King AC and Martin JE: Adherence to exercise. In *Resource Manual for Guidelines for Exercise Testing and Prescription.* Edited by American College of Sports Medicine. Philadelphia: Lea & Febiger, 1988.
12. Knapp DN: Behavioral management techniques and exercise promotion. In *Exercise Adherence: Its Impact on Public Health.* Edited by RK Dishman. Champaign, IL: Human Kinetics, 1988.
13. Martin JE and Dubbert PM: Behavioral management strategies for improving health and fitness. *J Cardiac Rehabil 4*:200–208, 1984.
14. Russell ML: *Behavioral Counseling in Medicine: Strategies for Modifying At-Risk Behavior.* New York: Oxford, 1986.
15. Sime WE and McKinney ME: Stress management applications in the prevention and rehabilitation of coronary heart disease. In *Resource Manual for Guidelines for Exercise Testing and Prescription.* Edited by American College of Sports Medicine. Philadelphia: Lea & Febiger, 1988.
16. Taylor CB and Miller NH: Basic psychologic principles related to group exercise programs. In *Resource Manual for Guidelines for Exercise Testing and Prescription.* Edited by American College of Sports Medicine. Philadelphia: Lea & Febiger, 1988.
17. Taylor CB, Miller NH and Flora J: Principles of health behavior change. In *Resource Manual for Guidelines for Exercise Testing and Prescription.* Edited by American College of Sports Medicine. Philadelphia: Lea & Febiger, 1988.
18. Wankel LM: Decision-making and social-support strategies for increasing exercise involvement. *J Cardiac Rehabil 4*:124–135, 1984.
19. Williams RL and Long JD: *Toward a Self-Managed Lifestyle,* 3rd Ed. Boston: Houghton-Mifflin, 1983.

CHAPTER 9

Program Administration

The administration of medically oriented programs for high risk or diseased patients differs from administration of health/fitness programs in a community, worksite, or university setting; yet, there are fundamental commonalities. Similarities exist in the knowledge base and skills required to operate the various types of programs by the Health Fitness Director (HFD) and the Rehabilitative Program Director (PD).

"Administrator" is a term unique to the public sector, universities, hospitals, and other non-profit entities. "Manager" is the term most often used in the private sector, including corporate facilities and commercial clubs. Manager, as a title, is becoming more common in hospitals as well. "Director" is yet another term that may be used. All of these titles refer to the individual who has as the primary responsibility the: (1) macro view (how the program fits into the organization as a whole), (2) program development, (3) program planning, (4) day-to-day operation, (5) program evaluation, and coordinating all aspects of the program.

THE MACRO VIEW

Mission Statement. The mission statement of the organization drives the program's development, planning, and ongoing operations, regardless of whether the health promotion setting is preventive or rehabilitative. The mission statement is a clearly defined, decisive and concise statement of the reason for the existence of the organization. It may often be referred to as the business prime objective.

Strategic Plan. The strategic plan, developed by top management, is a course of action laid out to achieve the mission statement or prime objective within a specified time period (e.g., 5 years). The objectives of the strategic plan directly relate to the success of the mission statement.

Goals, Objectives, and Action Plans. These are developed at the departmental level—the functional unit. They are short-term (usually 1 year) strategies and actions for the purpose of achieving the overall strategic plan and mission of the organization.

Figure 9–1 is an abbreviated example illustrating the relationships between the *mission statement,* developed by the Board of Directors, the *strategic plan,* developed by top management, and the *goals, objectives* and *action plans,* developed and implemented at the departmental level.

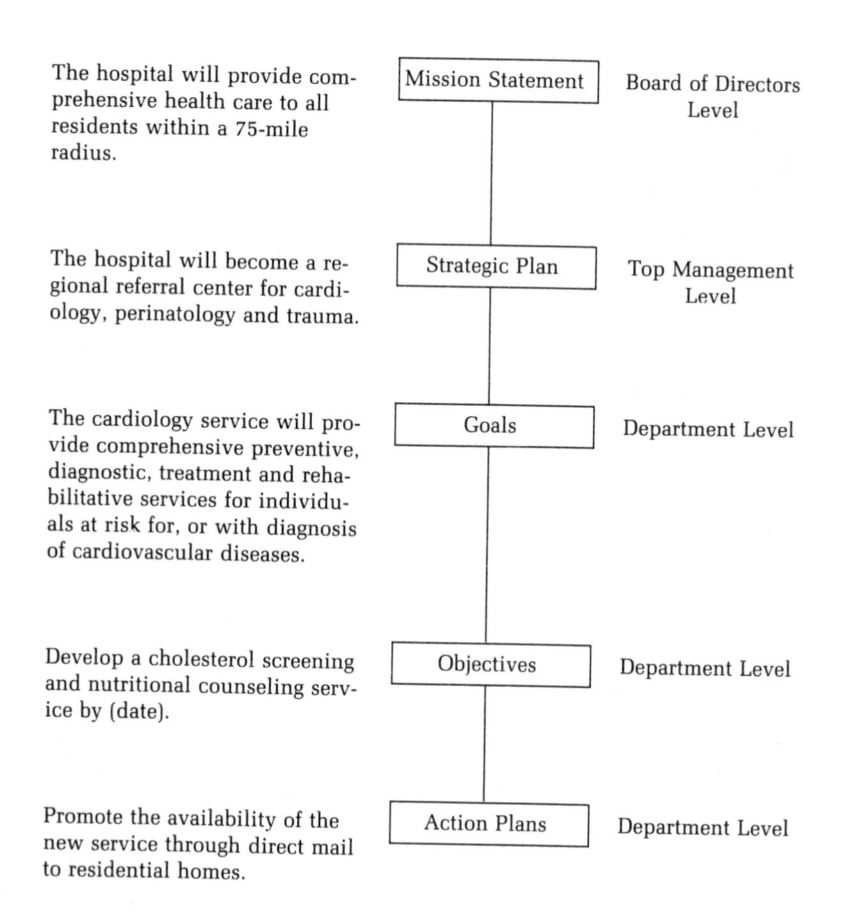

FIGURE 9–1.

Managerial Role. While there are many managerial or administrative functions, the HFDs/PDs can be succinctly described as individuals who manage themselves and the people who report to them, with the intent that both the organization and the consumer profit from the relationship. A major responsibility is to develop effective action plans to meet the goals and objectives of the department and be consistent with the strategic plan of upper management.

PROGRAM DEVELOPMENT

Structure and Organization. Carefully defined organizational relationships identify sources of authority, specific responsibilities, and lines of accountability. The HFD and PD have a strong professional knowledge base and skills, yet, each may be directly accountable to an individual with no background in the health/fitness or rehabilitative field. The HFD's/PD's primary accountability to this individual may include the areas of profit/loss, productivity, and pubic relations. Due to the complexity of rehabilitative and preventive programs, it may be necessary to establish an Advisory Board in order to address the problems encountered most effectively (see Fig. 9–2).

Facility Planning. Careful market analysis and volume projections, combined with a matching of program activities to facilities and equipment, will contribute to successful facility planning and program operation. At the same time, if projections indicate a need for facility expansion, new equipment, increased personnel, etc., then these findings would become a part of the next action or strategic plan.

Allocation of space and financial resources should be based on a thorough evaluation of the size of the target market and an estimation of projected market share. Careful attention must be given to patterns of client movement and hour-by-hour variations in client volume when planning the facility layout. Planning should include external factors such as parking and access, as well as internal factors, beginning from the time and location of participant registration and continuing, step by step, until the participant exits the facility.

Facility recommendations include: (1) exercise areas—walk/run track, aerobics room, weight training room, etc.; (2) exercise equipment—weight training, cycle ergometers, etc.; (3) educational areas—areas for group sessions, lectures, videos and written information, individual counseling area; (4) testing/evalu-

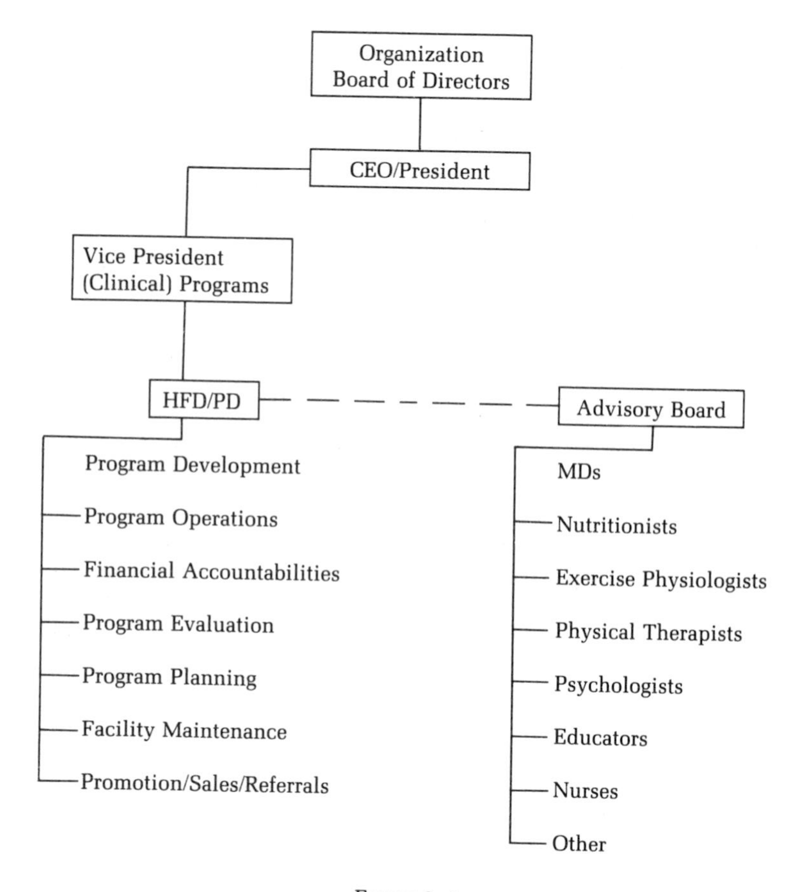

FIGURE 9–2.

ation area—quiet, private and offering easy access in case of an emergency; (5) business office/administrative area—secure records, staff work areas; (6) locker rooms and rest rooms; (7) emergency equipment area—secure but readily accessible to all areas of the facility.

Specific equipment requirements are determined by the types of programs offered, volume projections, and available capital resources. Special requirements for adequate ventilation and wet/dry areas for climatic situations should be addressed.

Personnel. The success of the program is closely tied to the selection of qualified personnel. Personnel qualifications include education, experience, and certification/licensure, as well as interpersonal skills of communication, motivation, and direction. A high level of technical skills and a strong knowledge base are important in the health/fitness and rehabilitative fields. However, in this environment significant emphasis is placed on leadership skills and the ability to provide examples and assist others with lifestyle changes.

Once the job functions are documented in written job descriptions, appropriate personnel are recruited. Here also, the specific personnel required are determined by the types of programs offered and resource limitations. The composition of the staffing may be the most significant distinction made between health/fitness programs and rehabilitative programs. Resource limitations may make it necessary to employ part-time personnel to address specialty needs of the program (i.e., nutritionists, physical therapists, etc.) or to rely upon the Advisory Board to a great extent.

Rehabilitative programs for clinical populations frequently employ nurses as the mainstay in staffing. Several states have written, and in some instances legislated, standards for cardiac rehabilitation programs that include requirements for staffing. All of these standards acknowledge the synergism of the multi-disciplinary approach to patient care. The multi-disciplinary cardiac rehabilitative team should minimally include: physician/medical director, certified program director, nurse(s), exercise physiologist(s), nutritionist(s), and behavioral psychologist. Other allied health professionals who may significantly enhance the quality and success of the program include respiratory therapists, physical therapists, occupational therapists, social workers, vocational specialists, and clergy.

Although the field of rehabilitative exercise science has evolved from several other professional disciplines, it now represents a new and separate body of knowledge. Due to the emerging nature of the field, many of the professionals involved draw on several specialties and/or advanced training and certification beyond their own specialty.

Health/fitness programs for apparently healthy individuals and for those with controlled disease depend on a somewhat different knowledge base and set of skills. However, personnel in this area also emerge from several types of training and backgrounds such as business, athletics, athletic training, adult fitness, sports medicine, physical education, nutrition, kinesiology, and exercise science. As in rehabilitative programs, the interdisciplinary training enhances program success and participant satisfaction in health/fitness programs.

The Business Plan. The business plan provides a rationale for financial needs, assists in raising capital, and helps in recruiting staff, as well as identifying staff needs. The start-up business plan differs from the annual or biennial business plan in that it: (1) requires significant allocation or reallocation of resources (capital); (2) provides an evaluation of the risks/benefits of the proposed *new program;* and (3) contains more detailed analysis and more speculative projections. The ongoing business plan contains the tactics of the long-range strategic plan that can be accomplished in 1 to 2 years with the intent of moving the organization toward the prime objective.

Many resources are available to assist the HFD/PD in business plan development. The most important function of a business plan is to evaluate ongoing performance and to identify areas that may require further analysis and modification of strategies.

Business plans may follow many different formats. Table 9–1 provides an outline of the components and their sequence common to most plan formats. The business plan format should be customized to fit the need of the proposed project or, in the case of an ongoing business plan, it should follow organizational guidelines.

PROGRAM PLANNING

Evaluation of Need. Program planning is an essential function of long-term program success. The effectiveness of the HFD/PD is enhanced by stepping back from the day-to-day operations and focusing attention on future needs of the program. Planning involves using the objective information from the program evaluation process combined with knowledge of industry trends and economics of the organization to determine need for program modification, redesign, growth or downsizing and/or enhancement (additional services).

The planning process must involve the participation and input of all personnel involved in the program. These individuals are vital in assisting with the development of action plans to achieve program goals and objectives. It is during the planning process that all obstacles to implementation of the plan should be identified and addressed. Involvement in the planning process ensures goal consensus, maintains momentum and generates enthusiasm.

Table 9–1. Components of the Business Plan

1. Summary
   Business Description
   - Name and location
   - Product/services
   - Market and competition
   - Management expertise

   Financial Needs Summary
   Operation Projections Summary
2. Description and History of Current Business
   - Brief history
   - Identification of need
   - Corporate mission and long range goals
   - Strengths, weaknesses, opportunities, and threats
3. Market Assessment
   - Description
   - Competition
   - Industrial trends
   - Market potential and customer base
   - Market strategy
4. Management
   - Key management personnel/experience
   - Board structure and role
   - Organizational chart
5. Technical and Operation Plan
   - General operating plan/policies
   - Costs/pricing
   - Critical risks and problems
6. Facilities
   - Rationale for location
   - Description
   - Leased/owned
   - Occupancy costs
7. Financial Plan
   - Capitalization plan
   - Explanation of financial structure
   - Summary/highlights of projected performance
   - Financial requirements/potential sources
   - Financial management

   Financial Statements (3-year projections)
   - Profit and loss statement forecasts
   - Proforma cash flow projections (by month)
   - Proforma balance sheets
   - Sources and uses of funds

   Explanation of financial projections
   - Best and worst case scenarios
   - Capital expenditure estimates
   - Strengths of plan
8. Appendix (optional)
   - Letters of support for concept
   - Market studies
   - Resumes of management team

Steps in Planning Process. The planning process involves the following steps: (1) define and describe the program as it currently exists, include all financial, market, quality and organizational information for the program evaluation process; (2) list alternatives and options; (3) describe in detail each alternative in terms of long-term and short-term goals, resource requirements, anticipated revenues, barriers to implementation, promotional needs, estimated expense budget, and timeline; (4) select the most promising alternatives and develop objectives; (5) consider strategies to reach objectives; (6) set a target date; (7) involve the participation of appropriate personnel; (8) define the performance objectives against which the program (new or modified existing) will be evaluated; (9) develop the business plan.

Implementation. Implementing the plan involves assigning the tasks, implementing the action plans, as well as supervising, coordinating and monitoring the action plans.

Thus, the management process begins again with collection and analysis of date from the operations process, evaluating the information from all appropriate sources, planning for improvement, and implementing the plan (see Fig. 9–3).

DAY-TO-DAY OPERATIONS

Managerial Responsibilities. Managerial responsibilities of the HFD/PD include supervisor, coordinator, teacher, evaluator, promoter, and planner. The director is responsible for: (1) the development and implementation of all program protocols and operating policies; (2) the coordination of services within the program to assure quality programming; (3) the hiring and supervising of all area/program managers and staff; (4) staff de-

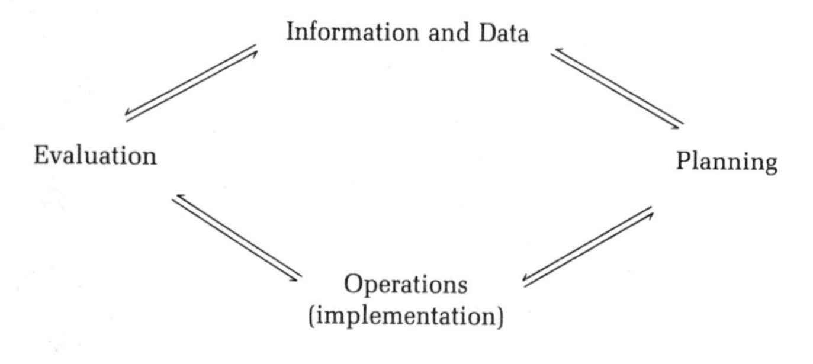

FIGURE 9–3.

velopment and staff training programs; (5) budget assessment, management of expenses, and recommendations to the Board of Directors for capital improvement/investments; (6) the coordination and approval of all promotional plans, marketing projects and public relations efforts; (7) program evaluation and planning for growth; (8) the development of research projects and the attainment of research funding; (9) the administration of testing and evaluation of participants; (10) the orientation and counseling of program participants. Although the HFD/PD is responsible for all aspects of the program, the magnitude of such a program may dictate that certain responsibilities be assigned to members of the staff.

Safety/Standards. The director is responsible for the development, implementation, and evaluation of all program policies and procedures. Organizations such as ACSM, American Association of Cardiovascular and Pulmonary Rehabilitation, American Heart Association, and several states have developed guidelines and checklists for quality assurance and control in rehabilitative and health/fitness programs. These resources should be used to develop, evaluate, and update program policies and procedures.

Most of these guidelines are not being used for external evaluation or accreditation, the exception being that some states have accreditation standards for cardiac rehabilitation. However, all hospital-based rehabilitative programming is subject to external audit by the Joint Commission on Accreditation of Hospitals (JCAH).

Policies and procedures should be documented in writing with citations of professional standards, state statutes, and other source documents. The attainment of safe and appropriate (patient) care (interaction) should serve as the main objective.[7] Program policies and procedures should be written under the advisement of medical, legal, and insurance professionals. The policies and procedures need systematic periodic review and updating.

Program policies and procedures should be written to cover such areas as: (1) emergency procedures—qualifications of personnel, assignment of duties during an emergency, equipment and supplies, updating and maintenance of equipment and supplies, drills and in-services, incident report procedures, communications (to paramedics, hospital personnel, etc.), audit mechanism for emergency team performance; (2) procedure for informed consent; (3) equipment safety/maintenance procedures; (4) personnel policies; (5) job descriptions and accountabilities; (6) participant grievance procedures; (7) evacuation procedures; (8) confidentiality policies; (9) procedure for assessment of eligibility for participation in program(s)—evaluation of health status, exercise testing, entrance criteria; (10) orientation procedure; (11) quality assurance audit procedure. The list is not meant to be all inclusive, but represents suggested guidelines for both Health/Fitness and Rehabilitative Programs. The Emergency Procedure is provided with more detail as an example for the development of all policies and procedures.

Legal Concerns. The recent emergence of the field of exercise science—both rehabilitative and health/fitness—has resulted in highly variable, nonstandard programs. The increasing numbers of individuals participating in some form of health/fitness program and the numbers of individuals at risk for cardiovascular, pulmonary, and metabolic disorders contributes to concerns over liability, proper insurance coverage, and medical clearance of participants. Hospital-based programs and all allied health and medical professionals are subject to various forms of peer review, government regulation, and association accreditation/certification. The health/fitness field is relatively unregulated and nonstandardized. Thus, the HFD/PD must look to the health care professions and to health/fitness professional associations for guidelines and standards that are reasonable and take into account that which is being done in similar settings. In the absence of specific regulations, litigation will be based on that which is reasonable, prudent, and consistent with policies and procedures in similar facilities such as hospital-based programs.

Proactive strategies of risk management will assist in minimizing the occurrence of legal problems such as: (1) careful screening and monitoring of participants; (2) properly obtaining informed consent; (3) written policies and procedures; (4) regular in-service and continuing education activities; (5) informing participants of program policies and guidelines; (6) thorough, real-time documentation of incidents.

PROGRAM EVALUATION

Program evaluation is an ongoing function that utilizes several sources of objective and subjective information. All programs must be systematically evaluated in terms of contribution to revenues, allocation of resources, cost, productivity, growth, public image, and continued strategic fit within the organization. Programs should be further evaluated in terms of services provided to the participant, family, and community.

The HFD/PD should utilize all sources of budgetary information and analysis to calculate total revenues, costs, productivity, and growth trends. Market surveys and consumer information polls are important sources of information regarding public perception of the program.

By defining measurable physiological, psychosocial and vocational goals for participants, an analysis can be conducted to quantify achievement of goals and thus evaluate the effectiveness of services provided to participants, families, and the community. The governing or advisory board of the organization can provide input regarding the ongoing strategic fit of the program with the ultimate decision being made by the Board of Directors and CEO.

Finally, a thorough analysis and review should be conducted regarding all incidents and incident reports. Recommendations and policy changes should be implemented to reduce or eliminate avoidable incidents and to improve the management of unavoidable incidents/emergencies.

Financial Accountability. The financial responsibilities and accountability of the HFD/PD are determined primarily by the organizational setting and the responsibilities provided by the CEO of the facility and program. However, a sound knowledge and understanding of financial management and budgetary process on the part of the director, enhances the success of any operation. Traditionally, the HFD/PD has not received academic training in the area of business management. Yet, realistic financial planning and goal setting are essential to the survival of any health/fitness or rehabilitative program. To enhance knowledge and experience in this area, the HFD/PD must draw on available resources from the organization if the program is within a hospital, university or corporate framework, and from methods used in small business management if the program is a free standing entity.

Minimally, the HFD/PD must have thorough understanding of budget preparation, how to monitor revenue and expenses, and how to understand the various financial statements appropriate in the setting. Furthermore, knowledge of accounting practices, employee benefits, taxes, and insurance enhance the effectiveness of the manager. No organization, large or small, can operate effectively without careful budget preparation and ongoing analysis. Budget preparation is, simply stated, projecting revenues and identifying and allocating costs. These are placed on a timeline and controlled (managed) to ensure cash flow and profitability.

The major source of income for health/fitness and rehabilitative programs are participant fees. These may be obtained directly from the participant or from health insurance carriers, Medicare, Worker's Compensation Funds, and/or vocational rehabilitation agencies. The HFD/PD must have a working knowledge of billing and collection procedures. The HFD/PD also benefits from an understanding of pricing and charge policies in effectively establishing rates for service.

Every effective manager must understand and control expenses to ensure profitability. Some guidelines for maintaining cost accountability include: (1) obtain and review all financial statements, review expense reports monthly; (2) set strategies and goals for expense management; (3) understand and tailor the chart of accounts to match program needs; (4) keep informed about potential cost increases; (5) obtain competitive bids for services and equipment; (6) understand industry trends in costs, charges and profitability.

REFERENCES

1. American College of Sports Medicine: *Resource Manual for Guidelines for Exercise Testing and Prescription.* Philadelphia: Lea & Febiger, 1988.
2. American Hospital Association: *Planning Hospital Health Promotion Services for Business and Industry.* Chicago, IL: American Hospital Publishing, 1982.
3. Blanchard MM and Tager MJ: *Working Well Managing for Health and High Performance.* New York: Simon & Schuster, Inc., 1985.
4. Blanchard K and Johnson MD: *The One Minute Manager.* New York: Wm. Morrow and Company, Inc., 1982.
5. Gerson RF: *Marketing Health/Fitness Services.* Champaign, IL: Human Kinetics, 1989.
6. Herbert WG and Herbert D: Legal aspects of cardiac rehabilitation exercise programs. *Phys Sportsmed 16*:105–111, 1988.
7. Hall LK and Meyer GC (Eds.): *Cardiac Rehabilitation: Exercise Testing and Prescription,* Vol II. Champaign, IL: Life Enhancement Publications, 1988.
8. International Racquetball and Sports Association: *Financial Management Manual.* Brookline, MA: IRSA, 1986.
9. Kotler P: *Marketing Management, Analysis, Planning and Control.* Englewood Cliffs, NJ: Prentice-Hall, Inc., 1980.
10. O'Donnel MP and Ainsworth T: *Health Promotion in the Workplace.* New York: John Wiley & Sons, 1984.

11. Patton RW, Corry JM, Gettman LR and Graf J: *Implementing Health/Fitness Programs.* Champaign, IL: Human Kinetics, 1986.
12. Patton RW, Grantham WC, Gerson RF and Gettman LR: *Developing and Managing Health/Fitness Facilities.* Champaign, IL: Human Kinetics, 1989.

CHAPTER 10

Program Personnel

Preventive and rehabilitative exercise programs for normal or at-risk populations can best be provided by a team approach. The composition of the team will be determined by the (1) population served, (2) location of the program, (3) number of participants, (4) availability of space and (5) availability of funding. The professionals assembled to deliver a preventive and/or rehabilitative exercise program may include a combination of the following: physicians: ACSM certified personnel such as exercise leaders, health fitness instructors, and directors; exercise test technologists, preventive and rehabilitative exercise specialists, and/or preventive and rehabilitative exercise program directors; dietitians, nurses, physical therapists, social workers, respiratory therapists, psychologists, and health educators. Certain members of the team may participate on a need or part-time basis.

Many individuals may benefit from a medical examination and an exercise stress test prior to entering into an exercise program. However, it is not necessary for everyone to do so (see Table 1–3). As the complexity of the preliminary testing and the risk level of participants increases, the composition of the personnel team will reflect greater responsibility. Exercise programs involving cardiac, pulmonary, renal, or other disease patients may well involve representatives from each of the specialty areas cited above.

PHYSICIANS

Physician involvement in all aspects of preventive and rehabilitative exercise programs is to be encouraged. Ideally, physicians should be involved from the earliest stages of program development. In developing a program, physicians should seek input from professionals from other disciplines who will be involved in the day-to-day operations of the program. In programs in which physicians are only interested in providing a supporting role, a program may be initiated by an exercise program director, exercise specialist, health fitness instructor, or health fitness director. Depending upon the nature and scope of the program, initiation and development may be accomplished by an exercise program director or health fitness director with physician guidance being provided through the establishment of a medical advisory board.

It is beneficial in any exercise program for the physician to take a leadership role. The physician is responsible for policies and procedures regulating the safety and well-being of participants. Emergency procedures need to be established with staff training and rehearsal occurring on a regular basis. The physician will also function in the role of diagnostician, decision maker, teacher and counselor, as well as assist in public relations. It is essential that physicians recognize the professional skills and competencies, and work as part of a team with exercise program directors, exercise specialists, exercise test technologists, exercise leaders, health fitness instructors and directors, dietitians, psychologists, etc., and delegate appropriate responsibilities.

Many physicians have been certified as preventive and rehabilitative program directors and as exercise specialists, but certification is not considered a necessary prerequisite for those who wish to assume medical direction of programs. The certification programs of the American College of Sports Medicine can evaluate the expertise and competence of a physician as a program director of a preventive or rehabilitative exercise program, but competence as a medical specialist is evaluated by the American Board of Medical Specialists and similar certifying organizations in other countries. Physicians involved in exercise programs must be licensed in that state to practice medicine and should be protected by professional liability insurance. They should maintain certification in advanced cardiac life support techniques or an equivalent (as the team emergency and safety leader).

Physicians have an important role in exercise testing, especially in higher risk, symptomatic, and diseased populations. Physicians involved in exercise testing need not be cardiologists or internists, but must be familiar with exercise testing procedures and the contraindications to exercise (see Table

4–1). Physicians must also be especially aware of effects of cardiorespiratory drugs on the ECG, as well as heart rate and blood pressure responses to exercise performance and training. The physician should be able to recognize ECG abnormalities and other physiological responses that may be encountered in exercise testing and dictate termination of an exercise stress test. These include such abnormalities as atrial and ventricular dysrhythmias, ST segment depression and elevation, left and right bundle branch block, AV block, and myocardial infarction.

Physicians should recognize the value of a maximal exercise test in the measurement of fitness, provision of information for exercise prescription, motivation of patients to exercise and diagnostic assessment for determining the likelihood of the presence of coronary disease. An exercise tolerance test can be an invaluable extension of a physical examination in detecting latent disease and assessing a patient's functional capacity. Physicians should be familiar with the various exercise protocols and how to select the appropriate protocol for the individual patient.

Physicians hold a unique position in teaching and motivating patients with regard to the benefits of exercise and other lifestyle modifications that may greatly enhance the quality of life. Physicians involved with exercise sessions and physicians in private practice who are not involved in group exercise programs may provide information and motivation to patients. Specific information should be provided such as frequency, intensity, duration, and progression of exercise rather than simply telling the patient to get more exercise. It is essential for the physician to provide follow-up on the exercise and encourage lifestyle changes during the medical follow-up in an effort to maintain the motivation of the patient and indicate the importance of these efforts. Physicians without interest or expertise in exercise training should seek qualified referral services in their communities in order to give their patients the benefit of appropriate exercise programming by trained, qualified individuals.

ACSM CERTIFIED PERSONNEL

The involvement of ACSM certified personnel in preventive and/or rehabilitative exercise programs is highly advisable because of the specific knowledge, skills, and competencies associated with each level of certification. There are two major categories of certification: the Health and Fitness Track and the Clinical Track. In previous editions of the *Guidelines for Exercise Testing and Prescription,* the Health and Fitness Track was referred to as the Preventive Track and the Clinical Track was identified as the Preventive/Rehabilitative Track. Although the overall mission of the respective tracks has not changed substantially, the names have been altered to better describe the primary audiences being served by personnel certified in these areas. The *Health and Fitness Track* is designed primarily for those who provide leadership in programs of a preventive nature for healthy individuals or those with controlled diseases in a corporate or community setting. The *Clinical Track* provides an added dimension which, in addition to providing leadership in programs of a preventive nature for healthy individuals or those with controlled diseases, also allows these personnel to work with diseased individuals enrolled in rehabilitative programs.

THE HEALTH AND FITNESS TRACK

With the Health and Fitness Track three levels of certification are offered:

Health Fitness Director
Health Fitness Instructor
Exercise Leader

Certification at a given level requires an individual to be knowledgeable about the behavioral objectives at that level and all levels below, as indicated in Table 10–1.

Exercise Leader (EXL)

Individuals certified at this level are considered to be "entry level" personnel who will serve under the leadership of a Health Fitness Instructor, Health Fitness Director, Exercise Specialist, or Program Director. The Exercise Leader's primary responsibilities in an exercise program are to demonstrate, lead, and explain proper exercise activities, as well as include pertinent information about precautions and safety. A fundamental knowledge concerning fitness for healthy individuals and those with controlled disease is required, as well as understanding basic motivation and counseling techniques.

It is recommended that candidates for Exercise Leader possess training credentials related to leading exercise, have at least

Table 10–1. Certification Levels and Behavioral Objective Requirements

Health and Fitness Tract			*Clinical Track*		
Exercise Leader (EXL)	*Health Fitness Instructor (HFI)*	*Health Fitness Director (HFD)*	*Exercise Test Technologist (ETT)*	*Preventive/ Rehabilitative Exercise Specialist (ESP)*	*Preventive/ Rehabilitative Program Director (PD)*
					PD
					ESP
				ESP	ETT
		HFD		ETT	HFD
	HFI	HFI		HFI	HFI
EXL	EXL	EXL	ETT	EXL	EXL

For example, an individual pursuing Exercise Specialist Certification must be able to demonstrate a thorough understanding of the behavioral objectives for the Exercise Leader, Health Fitness Instructor, Exercise Test Technologist, as well as the Exercise Specialist.

250 hours of hands-on leadership experience, or an academic background in exercise science, physical education, or an appropriate allied health field.

Health Fitness Instructor (HFI)

Certification at the level of Health Fitness Instructor requires a greater depth and breadth of knowledge in each of the areas encompassed by a multidisciplinary approach to health prevention of disease. The Health Fitness Instructor must demonstrate competence in exercise fitness testing, designing and executing an exercise program, leading exercise, and organizing and operating fitness facilities. The Health Fitness Instructor has the added responsibility of training and/or supervising Exercise Leaders during an exercise program and may serve as an exercise leader. In addition, the Health Fitness Instructor can serve as a health counselor to participants in need of multiple intervention strategies for lifestyle change.

Health Fitness Director (HFD)

The individual certified at this highest health and fitness level is required to have a command of the behavioral objectives of the two previous levels and will incorporate the administrative knowledge and skills as the director of a preventive program. The Health Fitness Director should have considerable background and experience with the administrative aspects of preventive programs, possess leadership qualities that ensure competence in the training and supervision of personnel, and be capable of program evaluation. Prior to obtaining the HFD certification, a candidate must be certified as a Health Fitness Instructor or Exercise Specialist.

THE CLINICAL TRACK

Within the Clinical Track, three levels of certification are offered:

Preventive/Rehabilitative Program Director
Preventive/Rehabilitative Exercise Specialist
Exercise Test Technologist

The title, "Clinical," indicates that personnel in this track are certified to provide leadership in health and fitness and/or clinical programs. Along with the knowledge and corresponding certification of the Health and Fitness Track, this group possesses the added clinical skills and knowledge which allow them to work with the higher risk, symptomatic populations. For example, if a person is certified at the Exercise Specialist level he/she is also certified at the Exercise Test Technologist, Health Fitness Instructor and Exercise Leader levels. Thus, an individual certified in the clinical track can provide leadership in preventive or rehabilitative programs at any level equal to or below the current level of certification (see Table 10–1).

Exercise Test Technologist (ETT)

The primary responsibility of the exercise test technologist is to administer exercise tests safely to individuals in various states of illness and health in order to obtain reliable and valid data. In addition, the exercise test technologist should demonstrate appropriate knowledge of functional anatomy, exercise physiology, pathophysiology, electrocardiography, and psychology in order to perform tasks such as preparing the exercise test station for administration of exercise tests, preliminary screening of the participant for the exercise test, administering tests and recording data, implementing emergency procedures when necessary, summarizing test data, and communicating the test results to the exercise specialists, program directors, and physicians. The exercise test technologist may administer an exercise test without a physician present based on the health status and age of the individual (see Table 1–3) or if the physician has provided clearance for the test. The technologist must be able to (1) recognize contraindications to exercise testing found in preliminary screening, abnormal responses during the exercise test and recovery, (2) respond appropriately, and (3) provide a summary of results.

Preventive/Rehabilitative Exercise Specialist (ESP)

The unique competency of the exercise specialist is the ability to lead exercises for persons with medical limitations, especially cardiorespiratory and related diseases, as well as to lead exercises for healthy populations. The exercise specialist (in conjunction with the program director or physician) has the knowledge to: design an exercise prescription based on the clinical state of the patient's results of an exercise test, evaluate participants' responses to exercise and conditioning, assist in the education of patients, and interact and communicate effectively with the physician, program director, exercise test technologist, program participants, and the community at large.

An exercise specialist is required to apply scientific principles of conditioning and motivating techniques for establishing a healthy lifestyle for individuals with medical or physical limitations. In all appropriately supervised exercise sessions, the goal should be to offer activities that will improve the participant's functional capacity, provide a variety of activities, and develop positive attitudes toward work and leisure.

Preventive/Rehabilitative Program Director (PD)

There is an increasing need to disseminate information about exercise testing, exercise prescription, and exercise programs to the medical and health-related professions and the general public. To meet this demand, an increasing number of qualified program directors are needed.

Program directors must have the knowledge and competencies of all other certification levels. In addition to the practical skills needed for exercise testing, prescription, and program development, program directors have a more extensive theoretical knowledge of medical and physiological implications of exercise testing and training. It is expected that the majority of this knowledge will have been obtained during studies for an advanced degree in fields such as exercise science, exercise physiology, physiology, medicine, nursing, physical therapy, or physical education.

Program directors are unique specialists in that they must draw from a wide range of abilities, knowledge, and experience as they relate to exercise. Program directors are responsible for: (1) developing appropriate screening procedures, including exercise testing; (2) developing individualized exercise prescriptions; (3) the administration, careful supervision and leadership of safe, effective and enjoyable exercise programs; (4) the implementation and supervision of lifestyle and behavioral change programs; (5) appropriate referrals to other disciplines; (6) education of the medical community, fitness community, patients and the general public about exercise and healthy lifestyle changes; (7) contributing, whenever possible, to research in the field of exercise and health.

With this combination of theoretical knowledge and practical experience, the program director should be capable of organizing and administering all types of programs. The program director should have the ability to plan and initiate new programs, reorganize and upgrade existing programs, work in programs for disease-limited patients and asymptomatic persons, as well as conduct research and explain its implications to personnel and clients.

The exact role of the program director depends on factors such as personnel involved, the size of the program, availability of funding, and participants involved. If the program is small, the program director may be involved in the hands-on activities of exercise testing and leadership. If the program is relatively large, then the duties may be primarily administrative and related to the actual prescription of the activity program in close cooperation with the physician. The program director's duties will also include the training, continuing education, and supervision of the other program personnel. Because of this, the program director should understand both the theoretical and practical aspects of exercise and conditioning. The program director needs to communicate the fundamentals of an exercise program in such a manner that it would enable the participant not only to improve physical condition, but also acquire a certain degree of autonomy in that improvement. For example, participants cannot always remain in a supervised, controlled exercise program. Thus, a program of continuing education is important so that the participants can continue to lead active, more healthful lives when they no longer desire or are unable to continue in a supervised program.

The program director is expected to integrate scientific principles of exercise physiology with pathophysiology and clinical medicine in order to deal with a wide variety of diseased individuals in prescribing exercise programs. Program directors are expected to keep abreast of new developments in the field by attending professional symposia, reading scientific articles and books, and by keeping in contact with professional organizations and colleagues. They are expected to inform and educate staff and physicians as to the significance of new developments. Program directors should continually strive to improve the level of competency within their specialty.

Administrative concerns that are major parts of diverse and complex preventive and rehabilitative exercise programs are another responsibility of the exercise program director. Issues such as involvement of specialized personnel, funding, third-party reimbursement, programming, liability, levels of medical supervision, staffing ratios, marketing, public relations are all a part of the program director's responsibilities.

OTHER PERSONNEL

The complexity and diversity of preventive and rehabilitative exercise programs demands that other specialized personnel be involved to some degree. The issues of available funding, specific client needs and programmatic direction will dictate the extent (part-time/full-time) and combination of personnel employed.

Each of the following provides certain benefits to an exercise program. For example, all programs can benefit from group presentations and individual counseling concerning foods and nutrition by a certified dietitian. Also, a health educator can assist in planning and delivering educational materials and lectures which will assist the client in developing a preventive, proactive style of living. A wellness manager, with a strong business background, is capable of providing not only fiscal management, but also programmatic development, advertising, and knowledge pertaining to wellness which extends beyond the realm of fitness.

Exercise programs that deal with rehabilitative populations may require additional personnel to address the special needs of the clients. Registered nurses, physical therapists, pulmonary therapists, social workers, psychologists, and occupational therapists have competencies which can strengthen the exercise program and enhance the rate of rehabilitation for the client. If the rehabilitative and preventive exercise programs are to achieve maximal results, the cooperation of the specialists interested in these programs must be used advantageously.

CHAPTER 11

Prerequisite Education and Work Related Experience for ACSM Certification

HEALTH AND FITNESS TRACK

Certification at a given level requires an individual to be knowledgeable about the behavioral objectives at that level and all lower levels (Table 10–1).

Exercise Leader. A fundamental knowledge concerning fitness for healthy individuals and those with controlled disease is required, as well as understanding basic motivation and counseling techniques.

It is recommended that candidates for exercise leader possess training credentials related to leading exercise, have at least 250 hours of hands-on leadership experience or an academic background in exercise science, physical education or an appropriate allied health field.

Health Fitness Instructor. The minimum educational prerequisite is a baccalaureate degree in exercise science, physical education or an appropriate allied health field or equivalent experience.

Health Fitness Director. The minimum educational prerequisite is a postgraduate degree in exercise science, exercise physiology, or an appropriate allied health field. Prior to obtaining the HFD certification, a candidate must be certified as a health fitness instructor or exercise specialist. In addition, in order to qualify as a health fitness director, an approved internship or period of practical experience of at least 1 year is required. The internship should be under the supervision of a certified program director and a physician, and provide opportunities to obtain competencies in administration, program leadership, laboratory procedures, and exercise prescription. It is assumed that the preceptor of the internship will work closely with the prospective health fitness director. In addition to the opportunity to demonstrate proficiency, oral and written examinations are an integral part of the learning experience.

CLINICAL TRACK

Certification at a given level requires an individual to be knowledgeable about the behavioral objectives at that level and all lower levels (Table 10–1).

Exercise Test Technologist. While there is no prerequisite experience or level of education required for the exercise test technologist, study in the fields of the biological sciences, medical technology, exercise science, physical education and health related professions are examples of appropriate training for those desiring certification. Although not mandatory, work experience under a physician or program director would be a valuable asset to the certification applicant. The certified exercise test technologist, working with individual participants during exercise testing and assisting in other roles in preventive and rehabilitative exercise programs, may gain the necessary experience to apply for the exercise specialist certification.

Preventive/Rehabilitative Exercise Specialist. The exercise specialist must possess a baccalaureate or master's degree in exercise science, nursing, physical education, or an appropriate allied health field. An internship of at least 6 months (800 hours) is required, largely with cardiopulmonary disease patients in a rehabilitative setting, with specific experience to obtain competency in the following areas:

a. Conducting and administering exercise tests
b. Evaluating and interpreting clinical data and exercise test results for the formulation of the exercise prescription
c. Conducting exercise sessions including the demonstration of leadership, proper monitoring, enthusiasm, and creativity
d. Responding appropriately to complications during exercise testing and training
e. Modifying the exercise prescription for patients with specific secondary limitations, beyond cardiopulmonary disease

Preventive/Rehabilitative Program Director. It is anticipated that an individual applying for certification will hold an advanced degree in a field such as exercise physiology, exercise science, physiology, medicine, physical education, or allied health related areas.

An internship or period of practical experience of at least 2 years is required. A significant amount of work with cardiopulmonary disease patients in a rehabilitative setting, with specific experience to obtain competency in the following areas is required:

a. Conducting and administering exercise tests
b. Evaluating and interpreting clinical data and exercise test results for the formulation of the exercise prescription
c. Conducting exercise sessions including the demonstration of leadership, proper monitoring, enthusiasm and creativity
d. Responding appropriately to complications during exercise testing and training
e. Modifying the exercise prescription for patients with specific secondary limitations, beyond cardiopulmonary disease
f. Involvement in administrative discussions and decisions
g. Involvement in evaluation of the program
h. Interaction with physicians and other rehabilitative team members

CHAPTER 12

General Objectives and Specific Learning Objectives for Exercise Program Certifications

Minimal competencies for each certification level have been outlined as behavioral objectives. A behavioral objective is a statement indicating what a person should be able to do following some unit of instruction or study. Two types of objectives are presented here. The General Objective (GO) describes the unobservable mental process, while the Specific Learning Objective (SLO) describes the behavior in observable terms.

Certification examination questions are constructed to test the individual's understanding of the information pertaining to the behavioral objectives. The ACSM publication, *Resource Manual for Guidelines for Exercise Testing and Prescription,* may be used to gain further insight pertaining to the topics identified by the behavioral objectives. It should be understood that the *Resource Manual* is not all-inclusive, nor is it intended to supplant the need to read the current literature. However, the *Resource Manual* may prove to be beneficial as a review of specific topics and as a general outline of many of the integral concepts to be mastered by those seeking certification.

As the level of certification increases, the depth of understanding and the knowledge base are expected to increase commensurately. Descriptive terms used in the behavioral objectives have been selected to reflect the level of difficulty and to help define the extent of knowledge one must possess to successfully qualify for certification.

For the entry levels of certification, the verbs "define," "identify," and "list" have been used. The midlevel certification behavioral objectives use "describe," "calculate," "plot," and "demonstrate," which imply the candidate must be able to deal with the knowledge base on a more sophisticated level. Being able to describe, demonstrate or mathematically manipulate principles, skills, or information reflects a greater understanding. The higher levels of certification demonstrate increasing complexity by using "discuss," "explain," "differentiate," "compare," and "teach." When the verbs "discuss," "demonstrate" and "teach" are used, the candidate must be prepared to interact with another person, such as on a practical examination or with the physician, patient, or client in the workplace. It is also implied that the candidate may be tested in written format with the understanding that the depth of knowledge and complexity of questions will be greater. Although the descriptive terms are generally stratified as described, they are not used exclusively at any level. For example, when appropriate, the descriptor "list" or "identify" may be used for one of the upper level behavioral objectives. Or, it may be equally appropriate to use "discuss" or "explain" at the lower level.

An individual pursuing certification is responsible for the behavioral objectives at that level and all lower levels (see Table 10–1).

BEHAVIORAL OBJECTIVES

The behavioral objectives for the six ACSM certification levels are provided below and are listed in the following order:

Health and Fitness Track

1. EXL
2. HFI
3. HFD

Clinical Track

1. ETT
2. ESP
3. PD

HEALTH AND FITNESS TRACK BEHAVIORAL OBJECTIVES

EXERCISE LEADER

Functional Anatomy and Biomechanics

EXL 01 GO 1

The candidate will demonstrate an understanding of human functional anatomy and biomechanics.

EXL 01 SLO 1

Describe the basic structures of bone, skeletal muscle, and connective tissues.

EXL 01 SLO 2
Describe the basic anatomy of the heart, cardiovascular system, and respiratory system.

EXL 01 SLO 3
Identify the major bones and muscle groups involved in gross human movement.

EXL 01 SLO 4
List and describe the actions of major muscle groups including trapezius, pectoralis major, latissimus dorsi, biceps, triceps, abdominal, erector spinae, gluteus maximus, iliopsoas, quadriceps, hamstrings, gastrocnemius, tibialis anterior.

EXL 01 GO 2
The candidate will demonstrate a knowledge of the role of biomechanical factors in the development of injuries.

EXL 01 SLO 5
Define the following terms: supination, pronation, flexion, extension, adduction, abduction, hyperextension, rotation, and circumduction.

EXL 01 SLO 6
Describe low back pain syndrome and describe exercises used to prevent this problem.

EXL 01 SLO 7
List and describe the types of joints in the body.

EXL 01 SLO 8
Describe the following abnormal curvatures of the spine: lordosis, scoliosis, and kyphosis.

EXL 01 SLO 9
Describe the biomechanical effects and potential risks of using hand/ankle weights.

EXL 01 SLO 10
Identify the interrelationships among center of gravity, base of support, balance, and stability.

EXL 01 GO 3
The candidate will describe common exercise movements and identify the major muscle groups involved in each.

EXL 01 SLO 11
Describe exercises designed to enhance muscular strength and/or endurance of specific major muscle groups.

EXL 01 SLO 12
Describe exercises for enhancing flexibility of major joints.

Exercise Physiology

EXL 02 GO 1
The candidate will demonstrate a knowledge of basic exercise physiology.

EXL 02 SLO 1
Define aerobic and anaerobic metabolism.

EXL 02 SLO 2
Identify the role of aerobic and anaerobic systems in the performance of various physical activities.

EXL 02 SLO 3
Define the following terms: ischemia, angina pectoris, tachycardia, bradycardia, myocardial infarction, cardiac output, stroke volume, lactic acid, hypertension, high density lipoprotein cholesterol (HDL-C), total cholesterol/high density lipoprotein cholesterol ratio, anemia, oxygen consumption, hyperventilation, hyperthermia, systolic blood pressure, diastolic blood pressure, isotonic, isometric, isokinetic, concentric and eccentric contraction, static and dynamic exercise, atrophy, hypertrophy, sets, repetitions, Valsalva maneuver, plyometrics.

EXL 02 SLO 4
Describe the role of carbohydrates, fats and protein as fuels for aerobic and anaerobic performance.

EXL 02 SLO 5
Describe the normal cardiorespiratory responses to an exercise bout in terms of heart rate, blood pressure and oxygen consumption. Describe how these responses change with adaptation to chronic exercise training and how men and women may differ in response.

EXL 02 SLO 6
Define and describe the relationship of METs and kilocalories to physical activity.

EXL 02 SLO 7
Describe the heart rate and blood pressure responses to static and dynamic exercise.

EXL 02 SLO 8
Identify the common sites and describe how heart rate is determined by pulse palpation. List precautions in the application of these techniques.

EXL 02 SLO 9
Calculate predicted maximal heart rate for various ages.

EXL 02 SLO 10
Identify the physiological principles related to warm-up and cool-down.

EXL 02 GO 2
The candidate will demonstrate an understanding of the basic principles involved in muscular strength, endurance, and flexibility training.

EXL 02 SLO 11
Identify the physiological principles related to muscular endurance and strength training: define overload, specificity of exercise conditioning, use-disuse, and progressive resistance.

EXL 02 SLO 12
List the physiological adaptations associated with strength training.

EXL 02 SLO 13
Describe the common theories of muscle fatigue and delayed muscle soreness.

EXL 02 SLO 14
Define the major components of physical fitness: flexibility, cardiovascular fitness, muscular strength, muscular endurance and body composition.

EXL 02 SLO 15
Define the major components of motor fitness: agility, speed, balance, coordination, and power.

EXL 02 SLO 16
Discuss the interrelationship of heart rate, exercise intensity, and O_2 utilization.

EXL 02 SLO 17
List the effects of temperature, humidity, altitude, and pollution upon the physiological response to exercise.

EXL 02 SLO 18
Identify the physical and physiological signs of over exercise, overtraining and overuse.

Human Development/Aging

EXL 03 GO 1
The candidate will demonstrate an understanding of the special problems of human development and aging.

EXL 03 SLO 1
Describe the changes that occur in maturation from childhood to older adulthood for the following areas: skeletal muscle, bone structure, reaction and movement time, coordination, tolerance to hot and cold environments, maximal oxygen consumption, strength, flexibility, body composition, resting and maximal heart rate, and resting and maximal blood pressure.

EXL 03 SLO 2
List the precautions associated with resistance and endurance training in youth and children. Explain how an exercise program could be modified to avoid aggravation of these problems.

EXL 03 SLO 3
Identity precautions associated with resistance and endurance training in the elderly. Explain how an exercise program could be modified to avoid aggravation of these problems.

EXL 03 SLO 4
Identify psychological factors frequently observed in the elderly (i.e., social withdrawal and adhering to developed habits).

Human Behavior/Psychology

EXL 04 GO 1
List several motivational techniques used to promote behavior change in the initiation, adherence or return to exercise and other healthy lifestyle behaviors.

EXL 04 SLO 2
List several teaching techniques used in the conduct of group or individual exercise programs.

EXL 04 SLO 3
List several techniques to deal with disruptive individuals in group programs (e.g., noncomplier, comedian, chronic complainer and the over-exerciser).

EXL 04 SLO 4
Define the psychological principles which are critical to health behavior change (i.e., behavior modification, reinforcement, goal-setting, social support and peer pressure).

EXL 04 SLO 5
Define and identify differences in Part versus Whole progressive learning theory as they relate to teaching exercise effectively in group or individual sessions.

EXL 04 SLO 6
Describe the personal communication skills necessary to develop rapport in order to motivate individuals to begin exercise, to enhance adherence and return to exercise.

EXL 04 SLO 7
Identify several techniques which can be used in an exercise program to facilitate skill development in muscular relaxation.

Pathophysiology/Risk Factors

EXL 05 GO 1
The candidate will identify risk factors which may require consultation with medical or allied health professionals prior to participation in physical activity.

EXL 05 SLO 1
Identify risk factors for coronary artery disease (CAD) and designate those that may be favorably modified by regular and appropriate physical activity habits.

EXL 05 SLO 2
Be familiar with the plasma cholesterol levels for various ages as recommended by the National Cholesterol Education Program.

EXL 05 SLO 3
Identify the following cardiovascular risk factors or conditions which may require consultation with medical or allied health professionals prior to participation in physical activity or prior to a major increase in physical activity intensities and habits: inappropriate resting, exercise and recovery HR's and BP's; new discomfort or changes in the pattern of discomfort in the chest area, neck, shoulder or arm with exercise or at rest; heart murmurs; myocardial infarction; fainting or dizzy spells; claudication; ischemia; cigarette smoking or other tobacco use; lipoprotein profile.

EXL 05 SLO 4
Identify the following respiratory risk factors which may require consultation with medical professionals prior to participation in physical activity or prior to major increases in physical activity intensities and habits: extreme breathlessness after mild exertion or during sleep, asthma, exercise-induced asthma, bronchitis, emphysema.

EXL 05 SLO 5
Identify the following metabolic risk factors which may require consultation with medical professionals prior to participation in physical activity or prior to major increases in physical activity intensities and habits: body weight more than 20% above optimal, thyroid disease, diabetes, or evidence of impaired carbohydrate metabolism.

EXL 05 SLO 6
Identify the following musculoskeletal risk factors which may require consultation with medical professionals prior to physical activity or prior to major increases in physical activity intensities and habits: osteoarthritis, rheumatoid arthritis, acute or chronic low back pain, prosthesis-artificial joints.

Health Appraisal and Fitness Testing

EXL 06 GO 1
The candidate will demonstrate and identify appropriate techniques for health appraisal and use of fitness evaluations.

EXL 06 SLO 1
Describe and demonstrate the use of health history appraisal to obtain information on past and present medical history, orthopedic limitations, prescribed medications, activity patterns, nutritional habits, stress and anxiety levels, family history of heart disease, smoking history, and use of alcohol and illicit drugs and know when to recommend medical clearance.

EXL 06 SLO 2
Describe the use of informed consent forms and medical clearances prior to exercise participation.

EXL 06 SLO 3
State the rationale for determining body composition.

EXL 06 SLO 4
Describe the types of tests for assessment of cardiorespiratory fitness, evaluation of strength, and flexibility, and techniques used to determine body composition.

EXL 06 SLO 5
Describe the difference between maximal and submaximal cardiorespiratory exercise tests.

EXL 06 SLO 6
Demonstrate the ability to measure pulse rate and blood pressure accurately both at rest and during exercise.

EXL 06 SLO 7
Identify the advantages and disadvantages of fitness participation.

EXL 06 SLO 8
Identify appropriate criteria for stopping an individual from exercising.

Emergency Procedures/Safety

EXL 08 GO 1
The candidate will demonstrate competence in basic life support and implementation of first aid procedures which may be necessary during or after exercise.

EXL 08 SLO 1
Possess current cardiopulmonary resuscitation certification or equivalent credentials.

EXL 08 SLO 2
Describe appropriate emergency procedures (i.e., telephone procedures, written emergency plan, personnel responsibilities. etc.).

EXL 08 SLO 3
Describe basic first aid procedures for heat cramps, heat exhaustion, heat stroke, lacerations, incisions, puncture wounds, abrasions, contusions, simple/compound fractures, bleeding/shock, hypoglycemia/hyperglycemia, sprains/strains, and fainting.

EXL 08 GO 2
The candidate will demonstrate an understanding of the risks associated with exercise participation.

EXL 08 SLO 4
Describe the reasons for not starting or terminating the exercise session.

Exercise Programming

EXL 09 GO 1
The candidate will demonstrate an understanding of the concepts of exercise.

EXL 09 SLO 1
State the recommended intensity, duration, frequency, progression and type of physical activity necessary for development of cardiorespiratory fitness in an apparently healthy population.

EXL 09 SLO 2
Differentiate between the dose of exercise required for various health benefits and that required for fitness development.

EXL 09 SLO 3
Describe the differences in an exercise program designed to develop versus one designed to maintain levels of cardiorespiratory fitness.

EXL 09 SLO 4
Describe the overload principle and how it relates to the exercise programming.

EXL 09 SLO 5
Identify and describe shin splints, sprains, strains, tennis elbow, bursitis, stress fracture, tendonitis, contusions, osteoporosis, arthritis, overweight, chondromalacia, blisters, skin irritations and lower back discomfort.

EXL 09 SLO 6
Define RPE and describe its relationship to metabolic responses to exercise and its role in exercise programming.

EXL 09 SLO 7
Demonstrate various methods for establishing appropriate exercise intensity and various methods for monitoring exercise intensity such as heart rate, and perceived exertion.

EXL 09 SLO 8
Describe the signs and symptoms of excessive effort which would indicate a change in the intensity, duration or frequency of exercise.

EXL 09 SLO 9
Describe and demonstrate aerobic exercise routines, class procedures and appropriate modifications in exercise programs which may be recommended by a physician for the following: elderly participants, participants of various fitness levels, acute illness (colds, etc.), controlled conditions such as exercise-induced asthma, allergies, hypertension, pregnancy and postnatal, obesity, and low back pain.

EXL 09 SLO 10
Demonstrate the ability to recognize common errors in body alignment and movement mechanics.

EXL 09 GO 2
The candidate will demonstrate an understanding of exercise for improving flexibility, muscular strength, and muscular endurance.

EXL 09 SLO 11
Describe the importance of flexibility and recommend proper exercises for improving range of motion of all major joints.

EXL 09 SLO 12
Describe and demonstrate exercises for the improvement of muscular strength and muscular endurance using various strength training techniques.

EXL 09 SLO 13
Define the following terms related to weight training methods: progressive resistance exercise, super-sets pyramiding, split routines, plyometrics, isokinetic, isotonic, isometric.

EXL 09 SLO 14
Identify isometric, isotonic, and isokinetic equipment.

EXL 09 SLO 15
List advantages and disadvantages of exercise equipment such as: stairmaster, rowing machines, mini-tramps, aerobic climber, heavy ropes.

EXL 09 SLO 16
Describe the hypothetical concerns and potential risks which may be associated with the use of exercises such as straight leg sit-ups, double leg raises, full squats, hurdlers' stretch, plough, back hyperextension, and standing straight leg toe touch.

EXL 09 GO 3
The candidate will demonstrate a knowledge of class organization and exercise leadership.

EXL 09 SLO 17
Describe and demonstrate appropriate exercises used in warm-up and cool-down for: aerobic conditioning classes, weight training, and sport participation (racket sports, volleyball, basketball, etc.).

EXL 09 SLO 18
Describe the difference between interval, continuous, and circuit training programs.

EXL 09 SLO 19
Demonstrate an understanding for the components incorporated into an exercise session and their proper sequence (i.e., warm-up, aerobic stimulus phase, cool-down, muscular endurance, and flexibility).

EXL 09 SLO 20
Recognize, analyze, and critique appropriate exercise class management and teaching techniques.

EXL 09 SLO 21
Describe signs and symptoms which indicate termination of exercise and physician consultation for a pregnant woman.

EXL 09 SLO 22
List various exercise class formations conducive to the following: leader visibility, participant interactions, exercise movement, leader communication.

EXL 09 SLO 23
Describe an exercise regimen for a water exercise class.

EXL 09 SLO 24
Describe partner resistance exercises that can be employed in a class setting.

EXL 09 SLO 25
Demonstrate a knowledge of techniques for accommodating various fitness levels within the same class.

EXL 09 SLO 26
Identify the differences between high impact and low impact aerobics classes and which class is appropriate for various participants.

Nutrition and Weight Management

EXL 10 GO 1
The candidate will demonstrate an understanding of the principles of weight management and nutrition.

EXL 10 SLO 1
Define the following terms: obesity, overweight, percent fat, lean body mass, anorexia nervosa, bulimia, and body fat distribution.

EXL 10 SLO 2
Discuss the relationship between body composition and health.

EXL 10 SLO 3
Compare the effects of diet plus exercise, diet alone, and exercise alone as methods for modifying body composition.

EXL 10 SLO 4
Describe the current misconceptions about spot reduction and rapid weight loss programs.

EXL 10 SLO 5
Explain the concept of energy balance as it relates to weight control.

EXL 10 SLO 6
Identify the functions of fat and water soluble vitamins and contrast their potential risk of toxicity with over-supplementation.

EXL 10 SLO 7
Discuss the inappropriate use of salt tablets, diet pills, protein powder, liquid protein diets, and other nutritional supplements.

EXL 10 SLO 8
Describe the importance of and procedures for maintaining normal hydration at times of heavy sweating and describe appropriate beverages for fluid replacement during and after exercise.

EXL 10 SLO 9
Demonstrate familiarity with the dietary guidelines recommended by the U.S. Department of Health and Human Services.

EXL 10 SLO 10
Identify the basic four food groups and give examples of food items found in each.

EXL 10 SLO 11
Describe the effects of diet and exercise on the blood lipid profile.

EXL 10 SLO 12
Describe the myths and consequences associated with inappropriate weight loss methods such as: saunas, vibrating belts, body wraps, electric muscle stimulators, and sweat suits.

EXL 10 SLO 13
List the number of kilocalories in 1 gram of fat, carbohydrate, protein, and alcohol.

EXL 10 SLO 14
Describe appropriate weekly weight loss goals.

EXL 10 SLO 15
Explain the set point theory of weight control.

HEALTH FITNESS INSTRUCTOR

Functional Anatomy and Biomechanics

HFI 01 GO 1
The fitness instructor will demonstrate an understanding of human functional anatomy and biomechanics.

HFI 01 SLO 1
Describe the structure and nature of movement that occurs in diarthrodial joints.

HFI 01 SLO 2
Describe the factors which determine range of motion in diarthrodial joints.

HFI 01 SLO 3
Describe the anatomy of the heart, respiratory, and vascular system.

HFI 01 SLO 4
Describe the biomechanical principles that underlie performance of the following activities: walking, jogging, running, swimming, cycling, lifting weights, and carrying or moving objects.

HFI 01 SLO 5
Describe the practical applications of the interrelationships among center of gravity, base of support, balance, and stability during physical activities.

HFI 01 SLO 6
Locate the common sites for measurement of skinfold thickness, skeletal diameters, girths for estimation of body composition; the anatomic landmarks for palpation of peripheral pulses; locate the bra-

chial artery and correctly place the cuff and stethoscope in position for blood pressure measurement.

Exercise Physiology

HFI 02 GO 1
The candidate will demonstrate a basic knowledge of exercise physiology.

HFI 02 SLO 1
Describe the primary difference between aerobic and anaerobic metabolism and their relative importance in exercise programs.

HFI 02 SLO 2
Describe the basic properties of cardiac muscle and the normal pathways of conduction in the heart.

HFI 02 SLO 3
Calculate the energy cost in METs and kilocalories for given exercise intensities in stepping exercise, bicycle ergometry, and during horizontal and graded walking and running.

HFI 02 SLO 4
Identify MET equivalents for various sport, recreational, and work tasks.

HFI 02 SLO 5
Discuss the physiologic basis of the major components of physical fitness: flexibility, cardiovascular fitness, muscular strength, muscular endurance, and body composition.

HFI 02 SLO 6
Explain the differences in the cardiorespiratory responses to static exercise compared with dynamic exercise, including possible hazards of static exercise.

HFI 02 SLO 7
Explain how the principle of specificity relates to the components of fitness.

HFI 02 SLO 8
Describe the physiological implications of warm-up and cool-down.

HFI 02 SLO 9
Describe the contributions of aerobic and anaerobic metabolism to energy expenditure at various exercise intensities.

HFI 02 SLO 10
Define and describe the implications of ventilatory threshold ("anaerobic threshold") as it relates to physical conditioning programs and cardiovascular assessment.

HFI 02 SLO 11
Explain the concept of detraining or reversibility of conditioning and its implications in fitness programs.

HFI 02 SLO 12
Discuss the physical and psychological signs of overtraining and provide recommendations to deal with these problems.

HFI 02 SLO 13
Describe the structure of the skeletal muscle fiber and the basic mechanism of contraction.

HFI 02 SLO 14
Describe the functional characteristics of fast and slow twitch fibers.

HFI 02 SLO 15
Explain contraction of muscle in terms of the sliding filament theory.

HFI 02 SLO 16
Explain twitch, summation, and tetanus in terms of muscle contraction.

HFI 02 SLO 17
Describe how each of the following differ from the normal condition: dyspnea, hypoxia, hypoventilation, orthostatic hypotension, premature atrial contractions, and premature ventricular contractions.

HFI 02 SLO 18
Describe blood pressure responses associated with changes in body position.

HFI 02 SLO 19
Define hypotension and hypertension and explain why blood pressure should be monitored during exercise testing.

HFI 02 SLO 20
List the physiologic adaptations to muscle metabolism and the cardiorespiratory system that occur at rest, during submaximal and maximal exercise following chronic aerobic training.

HFI 02 SLO 21
Describe the response of the following variables to steady state submaximal exercise and to maximal exercise: heart rate, stroke volume, cardiac output, pulmonary ventilation, tidal volume, respiratory rate, arteriovenous oxygen difference, systolic, diastolic, and mean blood pressure.

HFI 02 SLO 22
Describe the changes associated with chronic aerobic training for each of the variables: heart rate, stroke volume, cardiac output, pulmonary ventilation, tidal volume, respiratory rate, arteriovenous oxygen difference.

Human Development/Aging

HFI 03 GO 1
The health fitness instructor will demonstrate an understanding of the effect of the aging process on the structure and function of the human organism at rest, during exercise, and during recovery.

HFI 03 SLO 1
Characterize the differences in the development of an exercise prescription for children/youth, adult and older participants.

HFI 03 SLO 2
Describe special leadership techniques which might be used for children/youth and older participants.

HFI 03 SLO 3
Describe the unique adaptations to exercise training in children/youth and older participants with regards to strength, functional capacity, and coordination.

HFI 03 SLO 4
Describe common orthopedic and cardiovascular problems of older participants and what modifications in exercise prescription are indicated.

Human Behavior/Psychology

HFI 04 GO 1
The health fitness instructor will demonstrate an understanding of basic behavioral psychology, group dynamics and learning techniques.

HFI 04 SLO 1
Describe the specific strategies (e.g., operant conditioning) aimed at encouraging the initiation, adherence and return to participation in an exercise program.

HFI 04 SLO 2
Describe effective counseling communication skills in order to bring about behavioral change.

HFI 04 SLO 3
Describe how each of the following terms may impact upon the successful management of an exercise program: anxiety, depression, fear, denial, rejection, rationalization, aggression, anger, hostility, empathy, arousal, euphoria, and relaxation.

HFI 04 SLO 4
Discuss the potential manifestation of test anxiety (i.e., performance appraisal threat) during exercise testing and how it may disrupt accurate physiological responses to testing.

HFI 04 SLO 5
Describe the differential effects of exercise and progressive relaxation as stress management techniques for modifying anxiety, depression, anger, and for generating relaxation.

HFI 04 SLO 6
Discuss the behavioral change strategies which are appropriate or inappropriate for modifying body composition.

Pathophysiology/Risk Factors

HFI 05 GO 1
The health fitness instructor will demonstrate an understanding of the pathophysiology of the major chronic diseases and how these processes are influenced by physical activity.

HFI 05 SLO 1
Describe the atherosclerotic process and the risk factor concept.

HFI 05 SLO 2
Describe the role of physical activity in the prevention of atherosclerosis and hypertension.

HFI 05 SLO 3
Discuss the effect of regular physical activity on the lipoprotein profile and blood pressure.

HFI 05 SLO 4
Identify common drugs from each of the following classes and describe the principal action and the effects on exercise testing and prescription.

A. Antianginal (nitrates, beta blockers, calcium channel blockers, etc.)
B. Antihypertensive
C. Antiarrhythmic
D. Bronchodilators
E. Hypoglycemics
F. Psychologic stimulants

HFI 05 SLO 5
Identify the effects of the following substances on exercise responses: antihistamines, tranquilizers, alcohol, diet pills, cold tablets, caffeine, and nicotine.

Health Appraisal and Fitness Testing

HFI 06 GO 1
The candidate will demonstrate or identify appropriate techniques for health appraisal and use of fitness evaluations.

HFI 06 SLO 1
State the purpose and demonstrate basic principles of exercise testing.

HFI 06 SLO 2
Describe the categories of participants who should receive medical clearance prior to administration of an exercise test or participation in an exercise program.

HFI 06 SLO 3
Identify relative and absolute contraindications to exercise testing or participation.

HFI 06 SLO 4
Demonstrate the ability to obtain appropriate medical history, informed consent and other pertinent information prior to exercise testing.

HFI 06 SLO 5
Discuss the limitations of informed consent and medical clearances prior to exercise testing.

HFI 06 SLO 6
Demonstrate the ability to instruct participants in the use of equipment and test procedures.

HFI 06 SLO 7
Demonstrate the ability to assess flexibility, muscular strength, and muscular endurance.

HFI 06 SLO 8
Demonstrate various techniques of assessing body composition and discuss the advantages/disadvantages and limitations of the various techniques.

HFI 06 SLO 9
Discuss and demonstrate various submaximal and maximal cardiorespiratory fitness field tests using various modes of exercise and interpret the information obtained from the various tests including possible errors.

HFI 06 SLO 10
Discuss modification of protocols and procedures for cardiorespiratory fitness testing in children/youth.

HFI 06 SLO 11
Explain what physiological measures are taken during and after cardiorespiratory fitness testing and why.

HFI 06 SLO 12
Demonstrate the ability to interpret results of fitness evaluations on apparently healthy individuals and those with stable disease.

HFI 06 SLO 13
Describe and demonstrate techniques for calibration of a cycle ergometer and motor driven treadmill.

HFI 06 SLO 14
Identify appropriate criteria for discontinuing a fitness evaluation and demonstrate proper procedures to be followed after discontinuing such a test.

Emergency Procedures/Safety

HFI 08 GO 1
The health fitness instructor will demonstrate knowledge of emergency procedures, first aid, and evacuation plans.

HFI 08 SLO 1
Describe the emergency procedures, first aid, and evacuation plans needed during exercise testing, fitness evaluations, and exercise sessions.

HFI 08 SLO 2
Discuss the individual responsibility and legal implications related to first aid and emergency care.

HFI 08 SLO 3
Identify and maintain a safe environment for exercise testing and participation.

HFI 08 GO 2
The candidate will demonstrate an understanding of the risks associated with exercise testing.

HFI 08 SLO 4
Describe the risk of cardiovascular complications during exercise testing.

HFI 08 SLO 5
Discuss the risk factors for musculoskeletal injury and cardiovascular complications resulting from exercise training and how such risks might be reduced.

HFI 08 SLO 6
Identify the content and use of appropriate informed consent.

HFI 08 SLO 7
Explain the use of rest, cold, compression and elevation in the initial treatment of injuries, and the application of heat for long term treatment.

Exercise Programming

HFI 09 GO 1
The candidate will design and implement individualized and group exercise programs.

HFI 09 SLO 1
Describe and discuss the advantages/disadvantages and implementation of interval, continuous, and circuit training programs.

HFI 09 SLO 2
Design a program to increase strength using the various types of calisthenic exercises and equipment available.

HFI 09 SLO 3
Discuss the advantages/disadvantages of various commercial exercise equipment in developing cardiorespiratory fitness, muscular strength, and muscular endurance.

HFI 09 SLO 4
Describe special precautions and modifications of exercise programming for participation at altitude, different ambient temperatures, humidities, and environmental pollution.

HFI 09 SLO 5
Describe modifications in type, intensity, duration, frequency, progression, level of supervision, and monitoring techniques in exercise programs for patients with diabetes, obesity, hypertension, musculoskeletal problems, pregnancy/postnatal, and exercise-induced asthma.

HFI 09 SLO 6
Demonstrate an understanding for the components incorporated into an exercise session and their proper sequence (i.e., pre-exercise evaluation, warm-up, aerobic stimulus phase, cool-down, muscular endurance, and flexibility).

HFI 09 SLO 7
Describe the types of exercise programs available in the community and how these programs are appropriate for various populations.

Nutrition and Weight Management

HFI 10 GO 1
The candidate will demonstrate an understanding of the principles of weight management and nutrition.

HFI 10 SLO 1
Discuss guidelines for caloric intake for an individual desiring to lose or gain weight.

HFI 10 SLO 2
Calculate fat weight, fat free weight, and body weight at a specified percent body fat given current weight and percent fat.

HFI 10 SLO 3
Discuss the physiological effects of diet plus exercise, diet alone and exercise alone as methods for modifying body composition.

HFI 10 SLO 4
Describe the health implications of variation in body fat distribution patterns and the significance of waist/hip ratios.

HFI 10 SLO 5
Describe the caloric value of various physical activities as related to their potential role in weight loss programs.

HFI 10 SLO 6
Discuss how knowledge of an individual's overall health status and cardiac risk profile should be used in determining a recommended body weight.

HFI 10 SLO 7
Discuss the limitations of the various methods for measurement of body composition.

HFI 10 SLO 8
Demonstrate familiarity with the exchange lists of the American Dietetic Association, the N.I.H. Consensus Conference Statement on the health risks of obesity, the dietary recommendations of The American Heart Association and the A.C.S.M. position stand on proper and improper weight loss programs.

HFI 10 SLO 9
List six essential nutrients and describe the role of each.

HFI 10 SLO 10
List the common dietary sources of calcium and iron.

HFI 10 SLO 11
Describe the contraindications to very low calorie diets and the proper role of medical supervision in caloric restriction programs of various levels.

HFI 10 SLO 12
Explain the benefits and potential risks of protein sparing diets.

Program Administration

HFI 11 GO 1
The health fitness instructor will understand his/her supportive role in administration and program management.

HFI 11 SLO 1
Describe the documentation required when a client shows signs or symptoms during an exercise session which should be referred to a physician.

HFI 11 SLO 2
Demonstrate ability to create and maintain records pertaining to participant exercise adherence, retention, and goal setting.

HFI 11 SLO 3
Demonstrate ability to develop and administer educational programs, (i.e., lecture, workshops etc.) and materials (i.e., brochures, bulletin boards, etc.).

HEALTH FITNESS DIRECTOR

Functional Anatomy and Biomechanics

HFD 01 GO 1
The health fitness director will demonstrate a knowledge of human functional anatomy and biomechanics.

HFD 01 SLO 1
Discuss the relationship among biomechanical efficiency, oxygen cost of activity (economy), and performance of physical activity.

HFD 01 SLO 2
Discuss the applications of Newton's Laws of Motion to human movement.

Exercise Physiology

HFD 2 GO 1
The health fitness director will demonstrate a knowledge and a theoretical understanding of exercise physiology.

HFD 02 SLO 1
Discuss the functional and biochemical characteristics of fast and slow twitch muscle fibers.

HFD 02 SLO 2
Explain the concept of muscular fatigue during specific conditions of task, intensity, and duration of exercise.

HFD 02 SLO 3
Contrast the cardiorespiratory responses to acute graded exercise in conditioned and unconditioned subjects.

HFD 02 SLO 4
Given the absolute and relative levels of exercise intensity in conditioned and unconditioned individuals, compare the differences in cardiorespiratory responses.

Pathophysiology/Risk Factors

HFD 05 GO 1
The health fitness director will understand the interrelationship between acute and chronic disease conditions and physical activity.

HFD 05 SLO 1
Explain the risk factor concept of coronary artery disease (CAD) and the influence of heredity and lifestyle upon the development of CAD.

HFD 05 SLO 2
Explain the process of atherosclerosis, the factors involved in its genesis, and methods which may reverse the process.

HFD 05 SLO 3
Discuss in detail how lifestyle factors and heredity influence lipoprotein profiles.

HFD 05 SLO 4
Explain the causes of myocardial ischemia and infarction.

HFD 05 SLO 5
Explain the causes of hypertension, obesity, hyperlipidemia, diabetes, chronic obstructive and restrictive pulmonary diseases, arthritis, and gout.

HFD 05 SLO 6
Identify and explain the effects of the above diseases or conditions on cardiorespiratory and metabolic function at rest and during exercise.

HFD 05 SLO 7
Identify and explain the mechanisms by which exercise may contribute to preventing the above diseases.

HFD 05 SLO 8
Explain the use and value of the results of the exercise test and fitness evaluation for various populations.

HFD 05 SLO 9
Describe muscular, cardiorespiratory, and metabolic responses to exercise following a decrease in physical activity, bed rest, or casting of a limb for a period of 1 month.

HFD 05 SLO 10
Identify and discuss the causes and mechanisms of chronic obstructive pulmonary disease (COPD), exercise-induced asthma, and chronic asthma.

HFD 05 SLO 11
Identify current drugs from each of the following classes. Explain the principal action, and list the major side-effects.
A. Antianginal
B. Antiarrhythmic
C. Antihypertensive
D. Bronchodilators
E. Hypoglycemics
F. Psychologic stimulants
G. Vasodilators

HFD 05 SLO 12
Discuss the organization of a risk factor screening program, describe procedures, staff training, feedback, and follow-up.

Emergency Procedures/Safety

HFD 08 GO 1
The health fitness director will demonstrate competence in emergency procedures including the use, maintenance, and updating of appropriate emergency equipment, first aid supplies, and transport plans.

HFD 08 SLO 1
Provide instruction in the principles and techniques used in cardiopulmonary resuscitation.

HFD 08 SLO 2
Design and update emergency procedures for a preventive exercise program and an exercise testing facility.

HFD 08 SLO 3
List emergency drugs which should be available during exercise testing.

HFD 08 GO 2
The candidate will demonstrate the ability to create a safe environment for exercise testing and exercise participation.

HFD 08 SLO 4
Train staff in safety procedures, the epidemiology of risks of injury and cardiovascular complications, risk reduction techniques, and emergency techniques.

HFD 08 SLO 5
Describe the features of a safe exercise facility including environmental characteristics and appropriate policies.

HFD 08 SLO 6
Discuss the content of an informed consent document and other issues related to legal liability.

Nutrition and Weight Management

HFD 10 GO 1
The health fitness director will demonstrate an understanding of nutrition and weight management.

HFD 10 SLO 1
Discuss food preparation and presentation strategies which would promote heart healthy nutrition.

HFD 10 SLO 2
Compare the commercially available weight management programs.

Program Administration

HFD 11 GO 1
The health fitness director will understand the role of administration necessary for program and facility management.

HFD 11 SLO 1
Describe a management plan for the development of staff, materials for education, marketing, client records, billing, facilities management, and financial planning.

HFD 11 SLO 2
Describe a plan for the development, implementation and maintenance of first aid, and emergency procedures policies.

HFD 11 SLO 3
Discuss the components of a needs assessment/market analysis.

HFD 11 SLO 4
Discuss how each of the following affect the decision-making process: budget, market analysis, program evaluation, facilities, staff allocation, and community development.

HFD 11 SLO 5
Discuss the advantages and disadvantages of centralized versus decentralized management patterns.

HFD 11 SLO 6
Describe a personnel management plan including job description development, recruiting, interviewing, hiring, training, evaluation, procedures for professional advancement and termination of an employee.

HFD 11 SLO 7
Discuss strategies for managing conflict.

HFD 11 SLO 8
Discuss the development, evaluation and revision of policies and procedures for program components.

HFD 11 SLO 9
Describe and discuss the management-by-objective decision-making approach.

HFD 11 SLO 10
Describe personnel time management techniques for effective operation of a program.

HFD 11 SLO 11
Discuss the use of outside consultation: establishing contact, contracting for services and follow-up procedures.

HFD 11 SLO 12 Demonstrate an understanding of public relations strategies.

HFD 11 SLO 13
Identify the steps in development, implementation, and evaluation of a marketing plan.

HFD 11 SLO 14
Discuss various advertising techniques.

HFD 11 SLO 15
Demonstrate effective skills and techniques for communication, public speaking, and the use of audiovisuals for presentations to groups and individuals.

HFD 11 SLO 16
Diagram and explain an organizational chart and show the staff relationships between a health fitness director, governing body, medical advisor, and staff.

HFD 11 SLO 17
Identify and explain operating policies for preventive exercise programs including data analysis and reporting, reimbursement of service fees, confidentiality of records, relationships between program and referring physicians, continuing education of participants and family, legal liability, and accident or injury reporting.

HFD 11 SLO 18
Explain the legal concepts of tort, negligence, contributory negligence, liability, indemnification, standards of care, consent, contract, confidentiality, malpractice, and the legal concerns regarding emergency procedures and informed consent.

HFD 11 GO 2
The health fitness director will understand the principles of program evaluation.

HFD 11 SLO 19
Interpret applied research in the areas of testing, exercise, and educational programs in order to maintain a comprehensive and current state-of-the-art program.

HFD 11 SLO 20
Compare and contrast the various evaluation design models such as cross-sectional, longitudinal, case control and randomized clinical trials.

HFD 11 SLO 21
Discuss the establishment of a data base, including type of data to be collected, data management and analysis.

HFD 11 SLO 22
Discuss the elements of a program evaluation report.

HFD 11 GO 3
The health fitness director will understand principles of budget construction and management.

HFD 11 SLO 23
Describe the various revenue sources and their influence on short-term and long-term program planning.

HFD 11 SLO 24
Describe the steps in developing, evaluating, revising, and updating capital and operating budgets.

HFD 11 SLO 25
Describe the process of facility design and equipment selection and purchase.

HFD 11 SLO 26
Demonstrate an understanding of the different forms of a business enterprise such as sole proprietorship, partnership, corporation, and S-corporation.

CLINICAL TRACK BEHAVIORAL OBJECTIVES

EXERCISE TEST TECHNOLOGIST

Functional Anatomy and Biomechanics

ETT 01 GO 1
The exercise test technologist will demonstrate a knowledge of functional anatomy as related to exercise testing and fitness evaluation.

ETT 01 SLO 1
Locate the appropriate sites for the limb and chest leads for resting and exercise ECGs.

ETT 01 SLO 2
Locate the brachial artery and describe the cuff and stethoscope positions for blood pressure measurement.

ETT 01 SLO 3
Locate anatomic landmarks for palpation of peripheral pulses.

ETT 01 SLO 4
Locate common sites for measurement of skinfold thicknesses, widths, and girths.

ETT 01 SLO 5
Locate the anatomic landmarks used during cardiopulmonary resuscitation and emergency procedures.

Exercise Physiology

ETT 02 GO 1
The exercise test technologist will demonstrate a knowledge of exercise physiology.

ETT 02 SLO 1
Identify activities which are primarily aerobic or anaerobic.

ETT 02 SLO 2
List the cardiorespiratory responses associated with postural changes.

ETT 02 SLO 3
List physiological and clinical considerations in the selection of different modes of ergometry, i.e., treadmill, cycle, or arm ergometer.

ETT 02 SLO 4
Describe the principle of specificity as it relates to the mode of testing.

Human Development/Aging

ETT 03 GO 1
The exercise test technologist will demonstrate competence in selecting appropriate test protocol according to the age of the participant.

ETT 03 SLO 1
Describe adjustments which might be necessary for testing the younger and older participant, specifically, instructions for the patient and modification of the testing protocol and equipment.

Human Behavior/Psychology

ETT 04 GO 1
The exercise test technologist will demonstrate knowledge of psychological factors which may affect exercise test participants.

ETT 04 SLO 1
List six factors which increase anxiety in the exercise testing laboratory and describe how anxiety may be reduced in a participant.

ETT 04 SLO 2
List potential manifestations of test anxiety which can influence responses to an exercise test.

Pathophysiology/Risk Factors

ETT 05 GO 1
The exercise test technologist will demonstrate knowledge of the basic pathophysiology of ischemic heart diseases.

ETT 05 SLO 1
Define ischemia and list the methods that are used to measure ischemic responses. List the effects of ischemic heart diseases (including myocardial infarction) upon performance and safety during an exercise test.

ETT 05 SLO 2
List major risk factors for ischemic heart diseases.

ETT 05 SLO 3
Define normal blood pressure at rest and describe normal blood pressure responses to exercise and recovery. Explain why blood pressure should be monitored during the exercise test.

ETT 05 SLO 4
List special considerations necessary when testing participants with obesity, diabetes, renal disease, pulmonary disease, asthma, orthopedic problems, neurologic problems, hypertension, or stroke.

ETT 05 SLO 5
Recognize the drugs which may affect the ECG, heart rate or blood pressure at rest or during exercise (see Appendix B).

A. Antianginal (nitrates, beta blockers, calcium channel blockers, etc.)
B. Antiarrhythmic
C. Anticoagulant and antiplatelet
D. Lipid-lowering drugs
E. Antihypertensive (diuretics, vasodilators, etc.)
F. Digitalis glycosides
G. Bronchodilators
H. Tranquilizers, antidepressants, and antianxiety drugs

ETT 05 SLO 6
Define emphysema, asthma, chronic obstructive pulmonary disease, and psychogenic hyperventilation.

Health Appraisal and Fitness Testing

ETT 06 GO 1
The exercise test technologist will demonstrate the skills and knowledge for administering an exercise test.

ETT 06 SLO 1
Recognize inappropriate calibration of testing equipment and describe the need for calibration, i.e., a motor driven treadmill, cycle ergometer (mechanical), arm ergometer, electrocardiograph, aneroid and mercury column sphygmomanometer, and spirometers.

ETT 06 SLO 2
Perform a routine screening procedure prior to exercise testing, ensure informed consent is obtained, explain procedures and protocol for the exercise test, recognize the contraindications to an exercise test, and summarize and present screening information for the physician.

ETT 06 SLO 3
Identify patients for whom physician supervision is required.

ETT 06 SLO 4
Recognize the significance of patient history and physical exam findings as they relate to exercise testing.

ETT 06 SLO 5
Perform routine tasks prior to exercise testing including: taking a standard 12-lead electrocardiogram on a participant in the supine, upright, and post-hyperventilation conditions; accurately recording right and left arm blood pressure in different body positions; demonstrate the ability to instruct the test participant in the use of a rating of perceived exertion (RPE) scale and other appropriate subjective scales, such as dyspnea and angina scales.

ETT 06 SLO 6
Discuss the techniques used to minimize ECG artifact and the value of single-lead and multiple electrocardiographic lead systems in exercise testing.

ETT 06 SLO 7
Discuss the selection of the exercise test protocol in terms of modes of exercise, starting levels, increments of work, length of stages, frequency of physiologic measures.

ETT 06 SLO 8
Discuss how age, weight, level of fitness, and health status are considered in the selection of an exercise test protocol.

ETT 06 SLO 9
Contrast exercise testing procedures for pulmonary patients with that of cardiac patients in terms of exercise modality, protocol, physiological measurements, and expected outcomes.

ETT 06 SLO 10
Demonstrate appropriate techniques for measurement of physiological and subjective responses, i.e., symptoms, ECG, blood pressure, heart rate, RPE, and oxygen consumption measures at appropriate intervals during the test.

ETT 06 SLO 11
Recognize the need for modifying the testing procedures and protocol for children with clinical conditions.

ETT 06 SLO 12
Identify appropriate endpoints for exercise testing for various populations.

ETT 06 SLO 13
Discuss technical factors that may indicate test termination (e.g., loss of ECG signal, loss of power, etc.).

ETT 06 SLO 14
Discuss immediate post-exercise procedures and list various approaches to cool-down.

ETT 06 SLO 15
Record, organize and perform necessary calculations of test data for summary presentation to test interpreter.

ETT 06 SLO 16
Describe differences in test protocol and procedures when the exercise test involves radionuclide or thallium imaging procedures.

ETT 06 SLO 17
Demonstrate an ability to administer basic resting spirometric tests including FEV_1, FVC, and MVV.

ETT 06 SLO 18
Describe basic equipment and facility requirements for exercise testing.

ETT 06 SLO 19
Describe the responsibilities of the exercise test technologist on a typical testing day.

Electrocardiography

ETT 07 GO 1
The exercise test technologist will demonstrate knowledge of normal and abnormal resting ECGs and be able to recognize selected ECG abnormalities during exercise testing.

ETT 07 SLO 1
Describe the resting ECG by identifying important waves (P, QRS, T), segments (ST), intervals (PR, QRS, QT), and axis (QRS) which comprise the normal resting ECG.

ETT 07 SLO 2
Recognize changes in the ST segment, the presence of abnormal T waves and significant Q waves as well as their importance in resting and exercise ECGs.

ETT 07 SLO 3
Define the ECG criteria for terminating an exercise test due to ischemic changes.

ETT 07 SLO 4
Identify ECG patterns with the following conduction defects and dysrhythmias.

A. Identify ECG changes associated with the following abnormalities:
   1. Bundle branch blocks
   2. Atrioventricular blocks
   3. Sinus bradycardia (< 60) and tachycardia (> 100)
   4. Sinus arrest
   5. Supraventricular premature complexes and tachycardia
   6. Ventricular premature complexes (including frequency, form, couplets, salvos, tachycardia).
   7. Atrial fibrillation
   8. Ventricular fibrillation
B. Define the limits or considerations for terminating an exercise test based on the ECG abnormalities listed above.

Emergency Procedures/Safety

ETT 08 GO 1
The exercise test technologist will demonstrate competency in responding with appropriate emergency procedures to situations which might arise prior to, during, and after administration of an exercise test.

ETT 08 SLO 1
List and describe the use of emergency equipment which should be present in an exercise testing laboratory.

ETT 08 SLO 2
Demonstrate competency in verifying operating status of and maintaining emergency equipment.

ETT 08 SLO 3
Describe emergency procedures for a preventive and rehabilitative exercise testing program.

ETT 08 SLO 4
Possess current cardiopulmonary resuscitation certification or equivalent credentials.

EXERCISE SPECIALIST

Functional Anatomy and Biomechanics

ESP 01 GO 1
The exercise specialist will understand the biomechanical factors associated with various disease states, neuromuscular disorders, and orthopedic problems.

ESP 01 SLO 1
Discuss common gait abnormalities.

ESP 01 SLO 2
Discuss abnormal curvatures of the spine and their effects on the biomechanics of movement.

ESP 01 SLO 3
Discuss how muscular weakness and/or neurologic disorders affect the biomechanics of movement.

Exercise Physiology

ESP 02 GO 1
The exercise specialist will demonstrate an understanding of clinical applications of exercise physiology.

ESP 02 SLO 1
Describe the aerobic and anaerobic metabolic demands of various exercises for participants with cardiovascular, pulmonary and/or metabolic disease undergoing rehabilitation, and their implications.

ESP 02 SLO 2
Describe how each of the following varies for the healthy individual vs. the patient with coronary artery disease: function of the myocardium, the generation of the action potential, repolarization, and major variants in pathways of electrical activation.

ESP 02 SLO 3
Describe the cardiovascular responses to postural change before and after exercise testing.

ESP 02 SLO 4
List and be able to plot the normal resting and exercise values associated with increasing exercise intensity (and how they may differ for the coronary artery disease and/or COPD patient) for: heart rate, stroke volume, cardiac output, double product, arteriovenous O_2 difference, O_2 consumption, systolic and diastolic blood pressure, minute ventilation, tidal volume, and breathing frequency.

ESP 02 SLO 5
Discuss the potential hazards of isometric exercise for subjects with low functional capacities or patients with cardiovascular disease.

ESP 02 SLO 6
Describe the physiological effects of bed rest and discuss appropriate physical activities which might be used to counteract these changes.

ESP 02 SLO 7
Compare the unique hemodynamic responses of arm vs. leg exercise and of static vs. dynamic exercise.

ESP 02 SLO 8
Describe the determinants of myocardial oxygen consumption and the effects of exercise training on those determinants.

Human Behavior/Psychology

ESP 04 GO 1
The exercise specialist will demonstrate an understanding of basic behavioral psychology and group dynamics as they apply to crisis management, coping and lifestyle modifications.

ESP 04 SLO 1
Describe signs and symptoms of maladjustment/failure to cope during an illness crisis and/or personal adjustment crisis (e.g., job loss) that might prompt a psychological consult or referral to other professional services.

ESP 04 SLO 2
Describe the general principles of crisis management and factors influencing coping and learning in illness states.

ESP 04 SLO 3
Describe the psychological issues to be confronted by the patient and by family members of patients who have cardiorespiratory disease, and/or who have had an acute MI or surgery.

ESP 04 SLO 4
Contrast the psychological issues associated with an acute cardiac event vs. those associated with chronic cardiac conditions.

ESP 04 SLO 5
Describe the psychological stages involved with the acceptance of death and dying and recognize when it is necessary for a psychological consult or referral to a professional resource available in the community.

Pathophysiology/Risk Factors

ESP 05 GO 1
The exercise specialist will demonstrate an understanding of the cardiorespiratory and metabolic responses to increasing intensities of exercise in certain diseases and conditions.

ESP 05 SLO 1
Describe the cardiorespiratory and metabolic responses in myocardial dysfunction and ischemia at rest and during exercise.

ESP 05 SLO 2
Describe the cardiorespiratory and metabolic responses which accompany or result from pulmonary disease at rest and during exercise.

ESP 05 SLO 3
Describe the signs and symptoms of peripheral vascular diseases and the effects different kinds of exercise may have on each.

ESP 05 SLO 4
Describe the metabolic responses and possible complications of a diabetic patient at rest and during exercise.

ESP 05 SLO 5
Describe the influence of exercise on weight reduction, hyperlipidemia and diabetes.

ESP 05 SLO 6
Describe the effects of variation in ambient temperature, humidity, CO_2, and altitude on functional capacity and the exercise prescription. Explain required adaptations to the exercise prescription when environmental extremes exist.

ESP 05 SLO 7
Describe the etiology of atherosclerosis.

ESP 05 SLO 8
Describe the implications, symptoms, and mechanisms of classical and vasospastic angina.

ESP 05 SLO 9
Describe the methods used to measure ischemic responses.

ESP 05 SLO 10
Discuss the pathophysiology of the healing myocardium and the potential complications which may occur after an acute MI (extension, expansion, rupture, etc.).

ESP 05 SLO 11
Discuss *Risk Stratification* of patients after myocardial infarction. What materials are used and what are the prognostic indicators for high risk patients post MI.

ESP 05 SLO 12
Describe the effects of the following classifications of drugs on the ECG, heart rate and blood pressure. Also, list the common major symptoms of drug intolerance or toxicity in the following classes of medications (see Appendix B).

A. Antianginal (nitrates, beta blockers, calcium channel blockers, etc.)
B. Antiarrhythmic
C. Anticoagulant and antiplatelet
D. Lipid-lowering drugs
E. Antihypertensive (diuretics, vasodilators, etc.)
F. Digitalis glycosides
G. Bronchodilators
H. Tranquilizers, antidepressants, and antianxiety drugs

ESP 05 SLO 13
List the major effects of the above ten classes of drugs on physiologic responses and symptomatology, including ECG changes, at rest and during exercise testing and training.

ESP 05 GO 2
The exercise specialist will demonstrate an understanding of various modalities applied in the medical diagnosis and therapeutic management of certain diseases.

ESP 05 SLO 14
Describe the purpose and utility of coronary angiography, thallium perfusion scanning and radionuclide cineangiography.

ESP 05 SLO 15
Describe percutaneous transluminal coronary angioplasty (PTCA).

ESP 05 SLO 16
Describe the use of streptokinase and other thrombolytic agents.

Health Appraisal and Fitness Testing

ESP 06 GO 1
The exercise specialist will demonstrate competence in the interpretation of the exercise test for a rehabilitation program.

ESP 06 SLO 1
Describe the techniques used to calibrate a motor driven treadmill, cycle ergometer (mechanical), arm ergometer, electrocardiograph, aneroid and mercury column sphygmomanometer, spirometers, and respiratory gas analyzers.

ESP 06 SLO 2
Demonstrate appropriate techniques for measurement of oxygen consumption at appropriate intervals during an exercise test.

ESP 06 SLO 3
Modify testing procedures and protocol for children with clinical conditions.

ESP 06 SLO 4
Demonstrate the ability to provide objective recommendations to a patient following a cardiovascular event regarding physical conditioning, return to work and performance of selected activities of daily living (such as driving, stair climbing, sexual activity) based on exercise test results and clinical status.

ESP 06 SLO 5
Understand the prognostic implications of the exercise ECG and hemodynamic responses, thallium scintigraphy and radionuclide ventriculography and holter monitoring in post infarction risk stratification. Use this information in determining the appropriate setting for exercise, level of supervision, and level of monitoring.

Electrocardiography

ESP 07 GO 1
The exercise specialist will demonstrate an understanding of the important ECG patterns at rest and during exercise in healthy persons and in patients with CAD, pulmonary diseases, and metabolic diseases.

ESP 07 SLO 1
Describe the electrophysiological events involved in the cyclic depolarization and repolarization of the heart.

ESP 07 SLO 2
Describe the ECG changes which are associated with myocardial ischemia, injury, and infarction.

A. Identify ECG complexes typically seen in acute subendocardial ischemia, epicardial injury, and acute and chronic transmural and subendocardial infarction.
B. Identify ECG changes which correspond to ischemia in various myocardial regions (inferior, posterior, anteroseptal, anterior, anterolateral, lateral).
C. Differentiate between Q-wave and non-Q-wave infarction.

ESP 07 SLO 3
Identify ECG changes which typically occur due to hyperventilation, electrolyte abnormalities and drug therapy (see Appendix B).

ESP 07 SLO 4
Identify resting ECG changes associated with diseases other than CAD (such as hypertensive heart disease, cardiac chamber enlargement, pericarditis, pulmonary disease, metabolic disorders).

ESP 07 SLO 5
Explain possible causes of ischemic ECG changes and various cardiac dysrhythmias. Explain the significance of their occurrence during rest, exercise, and recovery.

ESP 07 SLO 6
Identify potentially hazardous dysrhythmias or conduction defects that may be observed on the ECG at rest and during exercise and recovery. Explain what procedures would be followed in case of such dysrhythmias or conduction defects.

ESP 07 SLO 7
Identify the significance of important ECG abnormalities in designation of the exercise prescription and in activity selection.

ESP 07 SLO 8
Discuss the indications and methods for ECG monitoring during exercise testing and during exercise sessions.

ESP 07 SLO 9
Identify ECG patterns with the following conduction defects and dysrhythmias: fascicular blocks and atrial flutter.

Emergency Procedures/Safety

ESP 08 GO 1
The exercise specialist will demonstrate competence in responding with the appropriate emergency procedures to situations in rehabilitative settings which might arise prior to, during, and after exercise.

ESP 08 SLO 1
Describe the emergency response(s) to cardiac arrest, hypoglycemia, bronchospasm, and sudden onset hypotension.

ESP 08 SLO 2
Identify the emergency drugs which should be available in exercise testing and participation situations and describe the mechanisms of action.

Exercise Programming

ESP 09 GO 1
The exercise specialist will demonstrate an understanding of the implications of exercise for persons with coronary artery disease risk factors and for patients with established cardiovascular, respiratory, metabolic, or orthopedic disorders and demonstrate competence in executing individualized exercise prescription.

ESP 09 SLO 1
Discuss the level of supervision and level of monitoring recommended for various patient populations in exercise programs.

ESP 09 SLO 2
Prescribe appropriate exercise based on medical information and exercise test data including intensity, duration, frequency, progression, precautions, and type of physical activity.

ESP 09 SLO 3
Modify a patient's exercise program (type of physical activity, intensity, duration, progression) according to the current health status of the patient with the following conditions: immediate post-coronary artery bypass surgery, MI, PTCA, heart transplantation, COPD, diabetes, obesity, renal disease, and common orthopedic and neuromuscular conditions.

ESP 09 SLO 4
Discuss basic mechanisms of action of medications that may affect the exercise prescription: beta adrenergic blocking agents, diuretics, calcium channel antagonists, antihypertensives, antihistamines, tranquilizers, alcohol, diet pills, cold tablets, caffeine, and nicotine.

ESP 09 SLO 5
Discuss warm-up and cool-down phenomena with specific reference to angina and ischemic ECG changes, dysrhythmias and blood pressure changes.

ESP 09 SLO 6
Discuss the differences in the physiological responses to arm and leg exercise in cardiac patients.

ESP 09 SLO 7
Discuss the appropriate use of static and dynamic exercise by cardiac patients.

ESP 09 SLO 8
Design a program of strength training for cardiac patients.

ESP 09 SLO 9
Discuss modifications in monitoring of exercise intensity for various patient groups.

ESP 09 SLO 10
Discuss possible adverse responses to exercise in various patient groups and what precautions may be taken to prevent them.

ESP 09 SLO 11
Discuss contraindications to exercise as related to the current health status of the participant.

ESP 09 SLO 12
Given a clinical case study, devise supervised exercise programs for the first 6 weeks after hospitalization for post MI, post PTCA, and post coronary artery bypass surgery and for the 3 months following.

ESP 09 SLO 13
Identify characteristics which correlate or predict poor compliance to exercise programs.

ESP 09 SLO 14
Identify and describe the role of the various allied health professionals and the indications and procedures for referral necessary in a multi-disciplinary rehabilitation program.

PROGRAM DIRECTOR

Exercise Physiology

RPD 02 GO 1
The program director will be able to discuss the mechanisms by which functional capacity, cardiovascular, respiratory, metabolic, endocrine, and neuromuscular adaptations occur in response to physical conditioning programs.

Human Development/Aging

RPD 03 GO 1
Explain differences in overall policy and procedures for the inclusion of different age groups in an exercise program.

RPD 03 SLO 1
Discuss facility and equipment adaptations necessary for different age groups.

Human Behavior/Psychology

RPD 04 GO 1
The exercise program director will understand the need for psychological consultation and referral of individuals who exhibit signs of psychological disorders.

RPD 04 SLO 1
Describe community resources for psychological support and behavior modification and outline an example of a referral system.

RPD 04 SLO 2
Describe the observable signs and symptoms of psychological disorder secondary to cardiopulmonary disorder.

Pathophysiology/Risk Factors

RPD 05 GO 1
The exercise program director will demonstrate an understanding of the relationships between different disease states and rehabilitative therapy.

RPD 05 SLO 1
Explain the process of atherosclerosis including current hypotheses regarding onset and rate of progression.

RPD 05 SLO 2
Demonstrate an understanding of lipoprotein classifications and their relationship to atherosclerosis or other diseases.

RPD 05 SLO 3
Contrast the signs and symptoms in the pulmonary versus cardiac patient during exercise testing and exercise training.

RPD 05 SLO 4
Explain the diagnostic and prognostic value of the results of the graded exercise test for various populations.

RPD 05 SLO 5
Explain the diagnostic and prognostic value of the low level predischarge exercise test versus the symptom-limited test and the indications for use with CAD patients.

RPD 05 SLO 6
Identify and explain the mechanisms by which exercise may contribute to preventing or rehabilitating individuals with cardiovascular, respiratory or metabolic diseases.

RPD 05 SLO 7
The program director will demonstrate an understanding of the following drug classifications, explain the mechanisms of principal actions, and list the major side effects, including ECG changes at rest and during exercise (see Appendix B).

A. Antianginal (nitrates, beta blockers, calcium channel blockers, etc.)
B. Antiarrhythmic
C. Anticoagulant and antiplatelet
D. Lipid-lowering drugs
E. Antihypertensive
F. Digitalis glycosides
G. Bronchodilators

H. Hypoglycemics
I. "Mood" elevators, stimulants
J. Emergency medications

RPD 05 GO 2
The program director will demonstrate an understanding of the various diagnostic and treatment modalities currently used in the management of cardiovascular disease.

RPD 05 SLO 8
Describe coronary angiography, radionuclide perfusion (thallium), and ventriculography (technetium) studies, including the type of information obtained, sensitivity and specificity, and associated risks and indications for use.

RPD 05 SLO 9
Describe percutaneous transluminal angioplasty as an alternative to medical management or coronary artery revascularization surgery in CAD. Demonstrate an understanding of the indications for percutaneous transluminal coronary angioplasty in different subsets of CAD patients versus coronary revascularization surgery or management with medications.

RPD 05 SLO 10
Describe the use of streptokinase and tissue plasminogen activator in acute myocardial infarction.

Electrocardiography

RPD 07 GO 1
The program director will demonstrate the ability to identify ECG patterns and to discuss implications for exercise testing, exercise programming, prognosis and risk stratification.

RPD 07 SLO 1
Explain the diagnostic and prognostic significance of ischemic ECG responses or dysrhythmias at rest, during exercise, or recovery.

RPD 07 SLO 2
Explain the causes and means of reducing false-positive and false-negative exercise ECG responses.

RPD 07 SLO 3
Understand Baye's theorem as it relates to pretest likelihood of CAD and the predictive value of positive or negative diagnostic exercise ECG results.

RPD 07 SLO 4
Discuss the role of ECG exercise testing as it relates to radionuclide perfusion (thallium) and ventriculography (technetium).

Emergency Procedures/Safety

RPD 08 GO 1
The program director will be knowledgeable about appropriate emer-

gency procedures for situations in rehabilitative settings which might arise prior to, during, and after exercise.

RPD 08 SLO 1
Diagram an emergency response system and discuss minimum standards for equipment and personnel required in settings for rehabilitative exercise programs.

Program Administration

RPD 11 GO 1
The exercise program director will understand the role of administration as a means of program facilitation.

RPD 11 SLO 1
Diagram and explain an organizational chart and show the staff relationships between an exercise program director, governing body, exercise specialist, exercise test technologist, fitness instructor, medical director or advisor, and participant's personal physician.

RPD 11 SLO 2
Identify and explain operating policies for preventive and rehabilitative exercise programs.

RPD 11 SLO 3
Describe the role of the medical director, supervising physician, and referring physician in the program design and implementation; and describe the responsibility of the program director to these individuals.

RPD 11 SLO 4
Describe and explain strategies for enhancing the understanding of the role of rehabilitation on the part of the public, health care policy makers, health care providers, and medical community.

RPD 11 SLO 5
Discuss the development and implementation of the comprehensive patient care plan.

RPD 11 SLO 6
Discuss the role of the rehabilitative staff in the development and implementation of the comprehensive patient care plan.

RPD 11 SLO 7
Demonstrate the ability to justify the inclusion of a comprehensive rehabilitation program in the health care setting.

RPD 11 SLO 8
Describe the concept of risk stratification and its application to program administration.

RPD 11 SLO 9
Identify and explain operating policies for clinical exercise programs including data analysis and reporting, reimbursement of service fees, confidentiality of records, relationships between program and referring

physicians, continuing education of participants and family, legal liability, and accident or injury reporting.

RPD 11 SLO 10
Demonstrate the ability to develop and present a comprehensive business plan for the development of a hypothetical clinical program in a non-profit institution.

APPENDIX A

Informed Consent for a Health-Related Exercise Test (Sample)

1. Explanation of the Exercise Test
   You will perform an exercise test on a cycle ergometer or a motor-driven treadmill. The exercise intensity will begin at a level you can easily accomplish and will be advanced in stages depending on your fitness level. We may stop the test at any time because of signs of fatigue or you may stop when you wish because of personal feelings of fatigue or discomfort.
2. Risks and Discomforts
   There exists the possibility of certain changes occurring during the test. They include abnormal blood pressure, fainting, disorder of heart beat, and in rare instances, heart attack, stroke, or death. Every effort will be made to minimize these risks by evaluation of preliminary information relating to your health and fitness and by observations during testing. Emergency equipment and trained personnel are available to deal with unusual situations that may arise.
3. Responsibilities of the Participant
   Information you possess about your health status or previous experiences of unusual feelings with physical effort may affect the safety and value of your exercise test. Your prompt reporting of feelings with effort during the exercise test itself are also of great importance. You are responsible to fully disclose such information when requested by the testing staff.

4. Benefits to be Expected
   The results obtained from the exercise test may assist in the diagnosis of your illness or in evaluating what type of physical activities you might do with low risk of harm.
5. Inquiries
   Any questions about the procedures used in the exercise test or in the estimation of functional capacity are encouraged. If you have any doubts or questions, please ask us for further explanations.
6. Freedom of Consent
   Your permission to perform this exercise test is voluntary. You are free to deny consent or stop the test at any point, if you so desire.

I have read this form and I understand the test procedures that I will perform. I consent to participate in this test.

____
Signature of Patient

________________ ________________________
Date Signature of Witness

Questions: ____

Response: ____

Signature of Physician or Delegate ______________________

When the test is for purposes other than diagnosis or prescription, e.g., experimental interest, this should be indicated on the Informed Consent Form. Policy on Human Subjects for Research is available on request from the ACSM.

APPENDIX B

Medications Relative to Exercise Training and Testing

Part I. Drug Names

Generic Name	*Brand Name*
Beta Blockers	
Acebutolol	Sectral
Atenolol	Tenormin
Metoprolol	Lopressor
Nadolol	Corgard
Pindolol	Visken
Propranolol	Inderal
Timolol	Blocadren
Alpha and Beta Blockers	
Labetalol	Trandate, Normodyne
Nitrites and Nitroglycerin	
Isosorbide dinitrate	Isordil
Nitroglycerin	Nitrostat
Nitroglycerin ointment	Nitrol ointment
Nitroglycerin patches	Transderm Nitro, Nitro-Dur II, Nitrodisc
Calcium Channel Blockers	
Diltiazem	Cardizem
Nifedipine	Procardia, Adalat
Verapamil	Calan, Isoptin
Nicardipine	Cardene
Nitrendipine	Baypress
Digitalis	
Digoxin	Lanoxin
Diuretics	
Thiazides	
Hydrochlorothiazide (HCTZ)	Esidrix
"Loop" Furosemide	Lasix
Ethacrynic acid	Edecrin

Part I. Drug Names *Continued*

Generic Name	*Brand Name*
Potassium-Sparing	
Spironolactone	Aldactone
Triamterene	Dyrenium
Amiloride	Midamor
Combinations	
Triamterene and hydrochlorothiazide	Dyazide, Maxzide
Amiloride and hydrochlorothiazide	Moduretic
Others	
Metolazone	Zaroxolyn
Peripheral Vasodilators	
Nonadrenergic	
Hydralazine	Apresoline
Minoxidil	Loniten
Angiotensin-Converting Enzyme (ACE) Inhibitors	
Captopril	Capoten
Enalapril	Vasotec
Lisinopril	Prinivil, Zestril
Alpha Adrenergic Blocker	
Prazosin	Minipress
Terazosin	Hytrin
Antiadrenergic Agents Without Selective Blockade of Peripheral Receptors	
Clonidine	Catapres
Guanabenz	Wytensin
Guanethidine	Ismelin
Guanfacine	Tenex
Methyldopa	Aldomet
Reserpine	Serapasil
Antiarrhythmic Agents	
Class I	
IA	
Quinidine	Quinidex, Quinaglute
Procainamide	Pronestyl, Procan SR
Disopyramide	Norpace
IB	
Tocainide	Tonocard
Mexiletine	Mexitil
Lidocaine	Xylocaine, Xylocard
IC	
Encainide	Enkaid
Flecainide	Tambocor
Multiclass	
Ethmozine	Moricizine
Class II	
Beta Blockers	
Class III	
Amiodarone	Cordarone
Bretylium	Bretylol

Part I. Drug Names *Continued*

Generic Name	*Brand Name*
Class IV	
Calcium Channel Blockers	
Bronchodilators	
Methylxanthines	
Aminophylline	Theo-Dur
Sympathomimetic Agents	
Ephedrine	
Epinephrine	Adrenalin
Metaproterenol	Alupent
Albuterol	Proventil, Ventolin
Isoetharine	Bronkosol
Terbutaline	Brethine
Cromolyn sodium	Intal
Hyperlipidemic Agents	
Cholestyramine	Questran
Colestipol	Colestid
Clofibrate	Atromid-S
Dextrothyroxine	Choloxin
Gemfibrozil	Lopid
Lovastatin	Mevacor
Nicotinic acid (niacin)	Nicobid
Probucol	Lorelco
Other	
Dipyridamole	Persantine
Warfarin	Coumadin
Pentoxifylline	Trental

Part II. Effects of Medications on Heart Rate, Blood Pressure, Electrocardiographic Findings (ECG), and Exercise Capacity

Medications	*Heart Rate*		*Blood Pressure*	*ECG*		*Exercise Capacity*
	Rest	*Exercise*	*[Rest (R) and Exercise (E)]*	*Rest*	*Exercise*	
Beta blockers (including labetalol)	↓ *	↓	↓	↓ HR*	↓ ischemia†	↑ in patients with angina; ↓ or ↔ in patients without angina
Nitrates	↑	↑ or ↔	↓ (R) ↓ or ↔ (E)	↑ HR	↑ or ↔ HR ↓ ischemia†	↑ in patients with angina; ↔ in patients without angina; ↑ or ↔ in patients with congestive heart failure (CHF)
Calcium channel blockers						
Nifedipine	↑	↑	↓	↑ HR	↑ HR ↓ ischemia†	↑ in patients with angina; ↔ in patients without angina
Diltiazem	↓	↓	↓	↓ HR	↓ HR ↓ ischemia†	↑ in patients with angina; ↔ in patients without angina
Verapamil	↓	↓	↓	↓ HR	↓ HR ↓ ischemia†	↑ in patients with angina; ↔ in patients without angina
Digitalis	↓ in patients $\overline{w}$ atrial fibrillation and possibly CHF. Not significantly altered in patients $\overline{w}$ sinus rhythm		↔	May produce nonspecific ST-T wave changes	May product ST segment depression	Improved only in patients with atrial fibrillation or in patients with CHF
Diuretics	↔	↔	↔ or ↓	↔	May cause PVCs and "false-positive" test results if hypokalemia occurs	↔, except possibly in patients with CHF (see text)

Vasodilators						
Nonadrenergic vasodilators	↑ or ↔	↑ or ↔	↓	↑ or ↔ HR	↑ or ↔ HR	↔, except ↑ or ↔ in patients with CHF
α-Adrenergic blockers	↔	↔	↓	↔	↔	↔
Antiadrenergic agents without selective blockade of peripheral receptors	↓ or ↔	↓ or ↔	↓	↓ or ↔ HR	↓ or ↔ HR	↔
Antiarrhythmic agents						
Class I	↑ or ↔	↑ or ↔	↑ or ↔ (R) ↔ (E)	May prolong QRS and QT intervals	Quinidine may cause "false-negative" test results	↔
Quinidine						
Disopyramide						
Procainamide	↔	↔	↔	May prolong QRS and QT intervals	Procainamide may cause "false positive" test results	↔
Phenytoin						
Tocainide						
Mexiletine						
Encainide						
Flecainide						
Class II						
Beta blockers	(see previous entry)					
Class III						
Amiodarone	↓	↓	↔	↔	↔	↔
Class IV						
Calcium channel blockers	(see previous entry)					
Bronchodilators						
Methylxanthines	↑ or ↔	↑ or ↔	↔	↑ or ↔ HR; may produce PVCs	↑ or ↔ HR; may produce PVCs	Bronchodilators ↑ exercise capacity in patients limited by bronchospasm
Sympathomimetic agents	↑ or ↔	↑ or ↔	↑, ↔, or ↓	↑ or ↔ HR	↑ or ↔ HR	
Cromolyn sodium	↔	↔	↔	↔	↔	
Corticosteroids	↔	↔	↔	↔	↔	

Part II. Effects of Medications on Heart Rate, Blood Pressure, Electrocardiographic Findings (ECG), and Exercise Capacity *Continued*

Medications	*Heart Rate*		*Blood Pressure*	*ECG*		*Exercise Capacity*
	Rest	*Exercise*	*[Rest (R) and Exercise (E)]*	*Rest*	*Exercise*	
Hyperlipidemic agents	Clofibrate may provoke arrhythmias, angina in patients with prior myocardial infarction Dextrothyroxine may ↑ HR and BP at rest and during exercise, provoke arrhythmias, and worsen myocardial ischemia and angina Nicotinic acid may ↓ BP Probucol may cause QT interval prolongation All other hyperlipidemic agents have no effect on HR, BP, and ECG					↔
Psychotropic medications:						↔
Minor tranquilizers	May ↓ HR and BP by controlling anxiety. No other effects.					
Antidepressants	↑ or ↔	↑ or ↔	↓ or ↔	(see text)	May cause "false-positive" test results	
Major tranquilizers	↑ or ↔	↑ or ↔	↓ or ↔	(see text)	May cause "false-positive" or "false-negative" test results	
Lithium	↔	↔	↔	May cause T-wave changes and arrhythmias	May cause T-wave changes and arrhythmias	
Nicotine	↑ or ↔	↑ or ↔	↑	↑ or ↔ HR; may provoke ischemia, arrhythmias	↑ or ↔ HR; may provoke ischemia, arrhythmias	↔, except ↓ or ↔ in patients with angina

Antihistamines	↔	↔	↔	↔	↔	↔
Cold medications with sympathomimetic agents	Effects similar to those described in *Sympathomimetic agents,* although magnitude of effects is usually diminished					↔
Thyroid medications Only levothyroxine	↑	↑	↑	↑ HR; provoke arrhythmias; ↑ ischemia	↑ HR; provoke arrhythmias; ↑ ischemia	↔, unless angina worsened
Alcohol	↔	↔	Chronic use may have role in ↑ BP	May provoke arrhythmias	May provoke arrhythmias	↔
Hypoglycemic agents Insulin and oral agents	↔	↔	↔	↔	↔	↔
Dipyridamole	↑ ↔	↔	↓ ↔	↔	↔	↔
Anticoagulants	↔	↔	↔	↔	↔	↔
Antigout medications	↔	↔	↔	↔	↔	↔
Antiplatelet medications	↔	↔	↔	↔	↔	↔
Pentoxifylline	↔	↔	↔	↔	↔	↑ or ↔ in patients limited by intermittent claudication

*Beta blockers with ISA lower resting HR only slightly. ↑, increase; ↔, no effect; ↓, decrease.

†May prevent or delay myocardial ischemia (see text).

From American College of Sports Medicine: *Resource Manual for Guidelines for Exercise Testing and Prescription.* Philadelphia: Lea & Febiger, 1988.

APPENDIX C

Informed Consent for a Cardiac Outpatient Rehabilitation Program (Sample)

1. Explanation of Outpatient Cardiac Rehabilitation Program
   You will be placed in a rehabilitation program that will include physical exercises, educational activities, and other health-related services. The levels of exercise which you will undertake will be based on your cardiovascular response to an exercise test. You will be given clear instructions regarding the amount and kind of regular exercise you should do. Organized exercise sessions will be available on a regularly scheduled basis. Your exercise sessions may be adjusted by the exercise specialist in consultation with the exercise program director and physician, depending on your progress. You will be given the opportunity for re-evaluation with a graded exercise test ________ months after the initiation of the rehabilitation program, and ________ thereafter. Other retests may be recommended as needed.
2. Monitoring
   Your pre-exercise blood pressure will be monitored, as required. You agree to learn, monitor and record, as instructed by staff, your own pulse rate before, during, and after each exercise session: participant's agreement shown by initialing here ________. In addition, ECG monitoring of your exercise prescription will be performed during the formal exercise sessions, if judged appropriate by the supervising physician.

3. Risks and Discomforts
   There exists the possibility of certain changes occurring during the exercise sessions. These include abnormal blood pressure, fainting, disorders of heart beat, and in rare instances heart attack, stroke, or death. Every effort will be made to minimize those risks by the provision of appropriate supervision during exercise. Emergency equipment and trained personnel are available to deal with unusual situations that may arise.
4. Benefits to be Expected
   Participation in the rehabilitation program may not benefit you directly in any way. The results obtained may help in evaluating in which types of activities you may engage safely in your daily life. No assurance can be given that the rehabilitation program will increase your functional capacity although widespread experience indicates that improvement is usually achieved.
5. Responsibility of the Participant
   To gain expected benefits and promote your safety, you must give priority to regular attendance and adherence to prescribed amounts of intensity, duration, frequency, progression, and type of activity. To achieve the best possible care:
   A. *DO NOT* withhold any information pertinent to symptoms from the exercise specialist, nurse, physician, exercise program director, or other professional personnel.
   B. *DO NOT* exceed your target heart rate.
   C. *DO NOT* exercise when you do not feel well.
   D. *DO NOT* exercise within 2 hours of using tobacco products (try to stop such use altogether).
   E. *DO NOT* exercise within 2 hours after eating.
   F. *DO NOT* exercise after drinking alcoholic beverages.
   G. *DO NOT* use extremely hot water during showering after exercise (stay out of sauna, steam bath, and similar extreme temperatures).
   H. *DO* report any unusual symptom that you experience before, during, or after exercise, or that you notice in an exercising colleague.
   I. *DO* check in with the exercise specialist after showering/dressing before leaving the site. If you plan to use other facilities at the site, please indicate that you will be doing so to the exercise specialist. At that time you

must accept total responsibility for yourself, and exercise at your own risk.

J. *DO* follow, without exception, all recommendations made by staff concerning the limits on any exercise, weight control, or other health-related activities which you may be encouraged to do and document by recordings.

6. Use of Medical Records
   The information that is obtained during exercise testing and while you are a participant in the Cardiac Rehabilitation program will be treated as privileged and confidential. It is not to be released or revealed to any person except your referring physician without your written consent. The information obtained, however, may be used for statistical analysis or scientific purpose with your right to privacy retained.
7. Inquiries
   Any questions about the rehabilitation program are welcome. If you have doubts or questions, please ask us for further explanation.
8. Freedom of Consent
   Your permission to engage in the Rehabilitation Program is voluntary. You are free to deny any consent if you so desire, both now and at any point in the program.

   I acknowledge that I have read this form in its entirety or it has been read to me, and that I understand the Rehabilitation Program in which I will be engaged. I accept the risks, rules, and regulations set forth. I consent to participate in this Rehabilitation Program.

Questions: ______________________________

Response: ______________________________

____
Signature of Patient

______________________ ______________________
Date Signature of Witness

Signature of Physician or Authorized Delegate ______________

APPENDIX D

Metabolic Calculations

Introduction

The rate of energy expenditure ($\dot{E}$) during exercise is often assessed through indirect calorimetry by the measurement of the rate of oxygen consumption ($\dot{V}O_2$). Clinically this measurement often is not available. Therefore, there is a need for simple and reasonably accurate estimates of $\dot{E}$ (e.g., $\dot{V}O_2$, METs) during steady state exercise. Considerable confusion arises over terminology.* The physical functions of force, work and power which are described below relate to the mechanical aspects of ergometry (the measurement of "work"). These mechanical aspects of ergometry have metabolic equivalents. We are primarily concerned with the metabolic equivalents, since they relate to "how much" or "how hard" the exercise is in biologic terms. The "load" applied is the mechanical element that stimulates an increased metabolism (the metabolic equivalent) during exercise. The purpose of the equations which follow is to relate mechanical measures of work rates to their metabolic equivalents and vice versa. These estimates are appropriate for general clinical usage when using standard ergometric devices but may have limited applications in other settings.

Definitions

The terms presented below can be expressed in many different units. Mechanical or non-metabolic measurements are ex-

*The American College of Sports Medicine has published definitions of terms and units used in sports science. See *Medicine and Science in Sports and Exercise,* Information for authors revised June, 1984.

pressed in units of the Système International d'Unités (SI) in scientific writing. Although these units may not be the most understandable units clinically, they are preferred. SI units are starred (*) in the text.

1. Force (F): An accelerating mass ($F = m \times a$, where m = mass and a = acceleration). A weight is a force. It is a mass undergoing gravitational acceleration. Typical units of weight are pounds (lb), newtons (N),* kiloponds (kp), kilograms (kg). (A kilogram is really a unit of mass, but in common usage, it is used as a weight). Kilograms will be used throughout this section both for body weight and for the amount of weight applied to an ergometer. Strictly, one kilopond = one kilogram (mass) undergoing unit gravitational acceleration. Thus, we typically write "1 kg = 1 kp" and they are often used interchangeably.
2. Work (W): A force moving through a distance ($W = F \times d$, where d = distance). Typical units of work are kp·m, kg·m, ft·lb, N·m, and joules (J)*. The metabolic equivalent of work is the total energy expended (E) in performing the mechanical work. A typical unit of E is kcal (Calories).
3. Power (P): The rate at which work is being done ($P = W \cdot t^{-1}$‡ where t = time). Typical units of power are $kp \cdot m \cdot min^{-1}$, $kg \cdot m \cdot min^{-1}$, $J \cdot min^{-1}$ and watts (W).* The metabolic equivalent of power is the rate of energy expenditure ($\dot{E}$) that occurs in response to the imposed mechanical work rate or power. Typical units of $\dot{E}$ are METs and $\dot{V}O_2$. It is $\dot{E}$ with which we are most concerned clinically. Non-weight bearing activities (e.g. cycle ergometry) are measured in units of absolute power. Measures of *absolute* mechanical power include $kp \cdot m \cdot min^{-1}$, $kg \cdot m \cdot min^{-1}$ and watts.* *Absolute* measures of $\dot{E}$ are $kcal \cdot min^{-1}$, $l\ O_2 \cdot min^{-1}$ and $ml\ O_2 \cdot min^{-1}$. Weight bearing activities (e.g. jogging) are measured in units of relative power. *Relative* measures of $\dot{E}$ include MET and $ml\ O_2 \cdot (kg\ body\ weight)^{-1} \cdot min^{-1}$, which is usually written $ml \cdot kg^{-1} \cdot min^{-1}$. Note that relative measures of $\dot{E}$ are all expressed "per kg body weight."

*Preferred SI unit.

‡Please note: The notation $W \cdot t^{-1}$ is equivalent to W/t i.e. the superscript "-1" can be read as "divided by" or "per" as in work divided by time or work per unit time.

4. MET: A multiple of the resting rate of O_2 consumption ($\dot{V}O_{2rest}$). One MET equals $\dot{V}O_{2rest}$ which is approximately 3.5 $ml \cdot kg^{-1} \cdot min^{-1}$; it represents the approximate rate of O_2 consumption of a seated individual at rest. Thus, an individual exercising at 2 METs is consuming O_2 at twice the resting rate (i.e., 7 $ml \cdot kg^{-1} \cdot min^{-1}$), while an individual exercising at 10 METs is consuming O_2 at 10 times the resting rate (i.e., 35 $ml \cdot kg^{-1} \cdot min^{-1}$).

Conversions and Useful Relationships

Distance:
  1 mi = 1.6 km*
Speed:
  1 $mi \cdot h^{-1}$ = 26.8 $m \cdot min^{-1}$
Weight:
  1 kg = 1 kp = 9.8 N*
  1 kg = 2.2 lb
Work:
  1 kcal = 4.2 kJ*
  1 l $O_2 \cong$ 5 kcal
  1 kg·m $\cong$ 1.8 ml O_2
Power:
  1 watt* = 1 $J \cdot s^{-1}$ = 1 $N \cdot m \cdot sec^{-1}$
  1 watt* = 6.1 $kg \cdot m \cdot min^{-1} \cong$ 6.0 $kg \cdot m \cdot min^{-1}$
  1 MET = 3.5 $ml \cdot kg^{-1} \cdot min^{-1}$
  1 MET $\cong$ 1 $kcal \cdot kg^{-1} \cdot h^{-1}$
  1 MET $\cong$ 1.6 $km \cdot h^{-1}$†
  1 MET $\cong$ 1.0 $mi \cdot h^{-1}$†

Usage

Table D–1 summarizes the important steps in calculating the rate of whole body work for a variety of standard activities. Note that for each activity, there are three components of $\dot{E}$ to be considered: horizontal, vertical or resistive, and resting. Summing these individual components gives the total $\dot{E}$ output during that activity. These equations can be used to estimate steady state $\dot{E}$ as well as to calculate what combination of speed/grade or weight/rpm applied to the mode will yield a desired $\dot{E}$. The calculations are done in units of $\dot{V}O_2$ ($ml \cdot kg^{-1} \cdot min^{-1}$ or

*SI units
†for running on a horizontal surface

ml·min^{-1}). It is easiest to perform all calculations in these units and then convert to METs, SI units, or other units as appropriate for your final answer.

Cautions

Direct determination of oxygen consumption is the standard measure of the metabolic response to exercise. This measurement requires the use of a breathing valve for collection and analysis of expired air during exercise. The $\dot{V}O_2$ for a given level of exercise is highly reproducible in a given individual; however, studies indicate that the measured $\dot{V}O_2$ at any given running speed, walking speed/grade will vary between individuals by approximately 7%. $\dot{V}O_2$ for a given activity is relatively unaffected by the environment, except in the presence of factors that may alter the mechanical work of the activity such as wind, snow or sand.

Due to the difficulty in direct measurement of $\dot{V}O_2$, equations have been derived to estimate the metabolic equivalent of a given activity. This estimate of the $\dot{V}O_2$ (or METs) is valid primarily for steady state exercise. When used to determine the metabolic equivalent of non-steady state or maximal workrate, it must be recognized that the measured $\dot{V}O_2$ may differ from estimated for two reasons: 1) if a steady state is not yet reached, the measured $\dot{V}O_2$ is less than the estimated $\dot{V}O_2$ and 2) exercise at maximal and near maximal intensities involves both aerobic and anaerobic components, which will result in an over-estimated MET level due to the unknown contribution of the anaerobic component to the exercise. The use of these equations to estimate METs, despite the discussed problems, is typically used in clinical settings to indicate the metabolic response to exercise on a treadmill or cycle ergometer. These formulae only give estimates of $\dot{V}O_2$ or METs.

Estimated METs can be used as a guideline for exercise prescription of activities in a neutral environment. The metabolic response to a given exercise (e.g. jogging at 161 m·min^{-1}) against a wind (which increases the external work which must be performed) is higher than the same exercise performed on the treadmill in a neutral environment. The use of METs for activity prescription should, therefore, be used carefully. Subjects should know appropriate heart rates for the activity and should check their heart rate response regularly. This is especially important in patients with ischemic heart disease, since approximately 80% of the increase in myocardial oxygen demand with exercise in the non-failing heart is a result of the increase in heart rate. Thus, heart rate is a much better indicator than estimated MET level of the appropriate exercise intensity relative to the myocardial oxygen supply/demand status.

Estimation of METs is also advantageous in exercise testing to express the metabolic response to external work. This provides a way to compare various treadmill protocols which use various combinations of speed and grade. Evaluation of progress in an exercise program can also be assessed in the same individual using estimated max METs, bearing in mind the limitation of estimation of max $\dot{V}O_2$ outlined above. Finally, without properly calibrated equipment, or with rail-holding during treadmill exercise, calculated $\dot{V}O_2$'s or METs are inaccurate and unreliable.

Walking

$\dot{V}O_2$ can be estimated with reasonable accuracy for walking speeds from 50 to 100 $m \cdot min^{-1}$ (1.9 to 3.7 $mi \cdot h^{-1}$). The O_2 cost of horizontal walking is 0.1 $ml \cdot kg^{-1} \cdot min^{-1}$ per $m \cdot min^{-1}$ of horizontal velocity $\left(\frac{0.1\ ml \cdot kg^{-1} \cdot min^{-1}}{m \cdot min^{-1}}\right)$. The O_2 cost of vertical work is $1.8\ ml \cdot kg^{-1} \cdot m^{-1} = \left(\frac{1.8\ ml \cdot kg^{-1} \cdot min^{-1}}{m \cdot min^{-1}}\right)$. (See Table D–1, walking, comment #2.) Since we do not walk up a vertical treadmill, the component of vertical work done is estimated by multiplying the O_2 cost of vertical work by treadmill grade (as a fraction) and speed. The resting component is one MET which equals 3.5 $ml \cdot kg^{-1} \cdot min^{-1}$.

Although $\dot{V}O_2$ estimates for walking are relatively accurate for most speeds and grades, there are exceptions. For example, the formula is more accurate in estimating $\dot{V}O_2$ when the participant is walking up a grade than on the level. Underestimates of 15 to 20% are expected with level walking, and 5 to 8% with walking up a 3% grade. Also, children are less efficient in walking and running than adults. The walking formula underestimates the oxygen requirement by approximately 0.5 $ml \cdot kg^{-1} \cdot min^{-1}$ for each year of age below the age of 18 years. The walking formula is equally accurate for men and women across the adult age range.

Running/Jogging

$\dot{V}O_2$ can be estimated with reasonable accuracy for speeds in excess of 134 $m \cdot min^{-1}$ (5 $mi \cdot h^{-1}$) and even for speeds as low as 80 $m \cdot min^{-1}$ (3 $mi \cdot h^{-1}$) if the subject is truly jogging (not walking). The O_2 cost of horizontal running at a given speed is about twice that for walking since running generally is a less efficient process than walking at lower speeds. High speed walking (>134 $m \cdot min^{-1}$) is also less efficient than running at the same speed. The vertical component of running on the treadmill is different from treadmill walking. When running up small grades some of the vertical lift normally found in level running is used to accomplish grade work, reducing the O_2 cost of grade work. This can be effectively corrected by multiplying the vertical component of the treadmill running by 0.5. Again, the resting component must be included. Since the O_2 cost of grade running off the treadmill may not be reliably predicted, the equation does not apply to this activity.

Leg Ergometry

$\dot{V}O_2$ can be estimated with reasonable accuracy for work rates between 300 and 1200 $kg \cdot m \cdot min^{-1}$ (50 to 200 watts*). There is no horizontal component to cycle ergometry since the cycle is stationary. Except in the cases of extremely obese or slight individuals, the mechanical work rate or power of cycling is related to the set resistance and revolutions per min and is independent of body weight. Thus, a given person weighing 60 kg will have the same absolute $\dot{V}O_2$ (i.e., in $ml \cdot min^{-1}$) at a given mechanical power on the cycle ergometer as a person weighing 90 kg. However, if expressed relative to body weight (i.e., in METs or $ml \cdot kg^{-1} \cdot min^{-1}$), the lighter individual would have a greater relative $\dot{V}O_2$. The mechanical power (in $kg \cdot m \cdot min^{-1}$) is determined by the product of the weight applied (kg or kp), the distance this weight travels per revolution ($m \cdot rev^{-1}$) and the number of revolutions per minute ($rev \cdot min^{-1}$), or $kg \cdot m \cdot min^{-1} = kg \times m \cdot rev^{-1} \times rev \cdot min^{-1}$. This power term should ultimately be converted into SI units by using the relationship $1\ W = 6\ kg \cdot m \cdot min^{-1}$. It should be noted that two common ergometers, the Monarch and the Tunturi, travel 6 $m \cdot rev^{-1}$ and 3 $m \cdot rev^{-1}$, respectively. To fully account for the added frictional work in the ergometer, the O_2 cost of the vertical or resistive work (1.8 $ml \cdot kg^{-1} \cdot m^{-1}$) is augmented by 0.2 $ml \cdot kg^{-1} \cdot m^{-1}$ so that for cycle ergometry the O_2 cost of work against the applied load equals the sum of these two values or 2.0 $ml \cdot kg^{-1} \cdot m^{-1}$. The resting component of O_2 consumption (corrected for body weight) is again added to obtain the total $\dot{V}O_2$.

Arm Ergometry

$\dot{V}O_2$ can be estimated with reasonable accuracy for work rates between 150 and 750 $kg \cdot m \cdot min^{-1}$ (25 to 125 watts*). The same considerations that apply to leg ergometry apply to arm ergometry; however, different constants apply. The O_2 cost of the resistive component (3.0 $ml \cdot kg^{-1} \cdot min^{-1}$) is larger than seen with other modes. This is most likely due to the involvement of considerable accessory musculature to stabilize the upper body during arm ergometry. The resting component of oxygen consumption corrected for body weight is again added to obtain the total $\dot{V}O_2$. Since the relationship between a person's $\dot{V}O_{2max}$ with leg ergometry and arm ergometry may be weak, it is important to do arm ergometry on individuals whose major occupational or leisure activities involve arm vs leg work. Furthermore, since the heart rate response to arm ergometry exceeds that seen at the same submaximal work rate in leg ergometry and since peak heart rate is less in arm than leg ergometry, arm ergometry testing is important for exercise prescription where arm work comprises a substantial portion of the exercise program.

Stepping

$\dot{V}O_2$ of bench and stair stepping varies with stepping rate, step height, and whether the person is stepping up or down or both. The O_2 cost of the horizontal component of stepping equals about 0.35 $ml \cdot kg^{-1} \cdot min^{-1}$ per $steps \cdot min^{-1}$ or $0.35 \left(\frac{ml \cdot kg^{-1} \cdot min^{-1}}{steps \cdot min^{-1}}\right)$. The O_2 cost of the vertical component of stepping depends upon the stepping rate ($steps \cdot min^{-1}$), the step height ($m \cdot step^{-1}$), and whether the person is stepping up, down, or both. The O_2 cost of stepping down is about 1/3 that of stepping up, so for each complete cycle (up and down) the O_2 cost is 1.33 times the O_2 cost of stepping up alone. Since the O_2 cost of vertical work is $\frac{1.8\ ml \cdot kg^{-1} \cdot min^{-1}}{m \cdot min^{-1}}$, the vertical O_2 cost for up and down stepping is $(m \cdot steps^{-1}) \times (steps \cdot min^{-1}) \times 1.33 \times \left(\frac{1.8\ ml \cdot kg^{-1} \cdot min^{-1}}{m \cdot min^{-1}}\right)$. Note that stepping height must be in meters, not centimeter or inches. The resting component has been included in the horizontal and vertical components.

Miscellaneous Activities

Rope skipping is convenient and requires the expenditure of a large number of calories, but it is difficult to vary the intensity of work and may be inappropriate for the average sedentary American or the typical patient with ischemic heart disease. Skipping at 60 to 80 skips·min^{-1} requires approximately nine METs. Doubling the rate of skipping to 120 to 140 skips·min^{-1} increases the work rate to 11 to 12 METs. Furthermore, the heart rate response tends to be higher than expected at comparable MET levels for walking or running. Thus, even the lowest rate of skipping (60–80 skips·min^{-1}) requires a MET level close to the maximum METs of the typical sedentary adult. In addition, this high MET level and the exaggerated heart rate response would tend to preclude rope skipping as an activity by the average patient with ischemic heart disease.

It is also difficult to vary the intensity of effort during rebound running on a mini-trampoline, since stepping rate varies little while an individual maintains a "normal" rebound height. Rebound running at the average stepping rate of 60 steps·min^{-1} requires approximately five METs. Due to the low acceleration forces seen with this activity, it may be a recommended activity for those individuals with lower extremity injuries who require moderate rates of energy expenditure. Exercise heart rate is not a good estimate of exercise intensity during rebound running.

Swimming is another activity which is difficult to grade due to the large differences in stroke efficiency among individuals. Average heart rates at a given submaximal $\dot{V}O_2$ are about 20 b·min^{-1} lower (range 5–50 b·min^{-1}) in the water than on land for walking activities requiring the same $\dot{V}O_2$. This decreases myocardial oxygen demand; however, maximal heart rates may also be lower in the water. Thus, a training heart rate based on a treadmill test may be too high during swimming activities and may need to be reduced to protect against early fatigue.

The energy cost of outdoor bicycling is also difficult to predict because it varies with bicycle characteristics, speed, grade and wind resistance. Wind resistance is related to frontal surface area of the cyclist which is a function of body weight. Therefore, the absolute oxygen cost of cycling in the ambient environment will be greater for the heavier individual than for the lighter one, all other conditions being similar. This is different from what is seen in laboratory cycle ergometry where individuals of different weights will have similar rates of oxygen consumption under similar experimental conditions.

The energy cost of aerobic dancing is also difficult to quantitate. Low intensity dancing (e.g., walking through the routine without overhead hand motion) requires about 3.5 METs while medium intensity dancing requires about five METs and high intensity dancing requires about nine METs.

Calculations

Table D–1 gives a visual presentation of how metabolic calculations may be done. The table is intended to be used as a guide for calculating various components of the energy cost formulas. The examples that follow show how various components of the energy cost formulas can be calculated. Always pay attention to units. Always place the appropriate units next to each quantity. If your units do not cancel to give the appropriate units for your answers, either your approach or your answer is incorrect.

Example 1:

Calculate the $\dot{E}$ in units of $ml \cdot kg^{-1} \cdot min^{-1}$ ($\dot{V}O_2$) and METs of the following activity:

treadmill speed = 2.5 $mi \cdot h^{-1}$
treadmill grade = 12 %
subject weight = 175 pounds

a) convert speed to $m \cdot min^{-1}$; note that subject weight does not enter into this calculation

$$(2.5\ \cancel{mi} \cdot \cancel{h}^{-1}) \times \left(\frac{26.8\ m \cdot min^{-1}}{\cancel{mi} \cdot \cancel{h}^{-1}}\right) = 67\ m \cdot min^{-1}$$

(Note that the slashes indicate cancellation of units.)

b) calculate horizontal component (HC)

$$HC = (m \cdot min^{-1}) \times \left(\frac{0.1\ ml \cdot kg^{-1} \cdot min^{-1}}{m \cdot min^{-1}}\right)$$

$$= (67\ \cancel{m} \cdot \cancel{min}^{-1}) \times \left(\frac{0.1\ ml \cdot kg^{-1} \cdot min^{-1}}{\cancel{m} \cdot \cancel{min}^{-1}}\right)$$

$$= 6.7\ ml \cdot kg^{-1} \cdot min^{-1}$$

c) calculate vertical component (VC); note that grade must be a fraction

$$VC = (\text{grade}) \times (\text{m}\cdot\text{min}^{-1}) \times \left(\frac{1.8\ \text{ml}\cdot\text{kg}^{-1}\cdot\text{min}^{-1}}{\text{m}\cdot\text{min}^{-1}}\right)$$

$$= (.12) \times (67\ \text{m}\cdot\text{min}^{-1}) \times \left(\frac{1.8\ \text{ml}\cdot\text{kg}^{-1}\cdot\text{min}^{-1}}{\text{m}\cdot\text{min}^{-1}}\right)$$

$$= 14.5\ \text{ml}\cdot\text{kg}^{-1}\cdot\text{min}^{-1}$$

d) calculate $\dot{V}O_2$ in $\text{ml}\cdot\text{kg}^{-1}\cdot\text{min}^{-1}$

$$\dot{V}O_2 = (HC) + (VC) + \text{Rest}$$

$$= (6.7\ \text{ml}\cdot\text{kg}^{-1}\cdot\text{min}^{-1}) + (14.5\ \text{ml}\cdot\text{kg}^{-1}\cdot\text{min}^{-1}) + (3.5\ \text{ml}\cdot\text{kg}^{-1}\cdot\text{min}^{-1})$$

$$= 24.7\ \text{ml}\cdot\text{kg}^{-1}\cdot\text{min}^{-1}$$

e) calculate $\dot{E}$ in METs by converting $\dot{V}O_2$ to METs

$$\dot{E} = \dot{V}O_2 \times \left(\frac{1\ \text{MET}}{3.5\ \text{ml}\cdot\text{kg}^{-1}\cdot\text{min}^{-1}}\right)$$

$$= (24.7\ \text{ml}\cdot\text{kg}^{-1}\cdot\text{min}^{-1}) \times \left(\frac{1\ \text{MET}}{3.5\ \text{ml}\cdot\text{kg}^{-1}\cdot\text{min}^{-1}}\right)$$

$$= 7.1\ \text{METs}$$

Example 2

A subject has a maximal exercise capacity of 12 METs. The exercise prescription is for 70% of maximal capacity using a cycle ergometer. Calculate the mechanical power appropriate to obtain this prescribed level. The subject weighs 172 lb. Note: Our approach is to solve for the mechanical power term $\left(\frac{\text{kg}\cdot\text{m}}{\text{min}}\right)$ in the resistive component and convert to SI units. For clarity of illustration, this calculation has been split into its component parts.

a) convert lb to kg

$$(172\ \text{lb}) \times \left(\frac{1\ \text{kg}}{2.2\ \text{lb}}\right) = 78.2\ \text{kg}$$

b) calculate training METs

$$\dot{E} = 0.70 \times \dot{E}_{max}$$
$$= (0.70) \times 12 \text{ METs}$$
$$= 8.4 \text{ METs}$$

c) calculate training $\dot{V}O_2$ (in $ml \cdot kg^{-1} \cdot min^{-1}$)

$$\dot{V}O_2 = \dot{E}\ (\text{METs}) \times \left(\frac{3.5\ ml \cdot kg^{-1} \cdot min^{-1}}{1\ \text{MET}}\right)$$
$$= (8.4\ \text{METs}) \times \left(\frac{3.5\ ml \cdot kg^{-1} \cdot min^{-1}}{1\ \text{MET}}\right)$$
$$= 29.4\ ml \cdot kg^{-1} \cdot min^{-1}$$

d) convert relative $\dot{V}O_2$ to absolute $\dot{V}O_2$

$$\dot{V}O_2\ (ml \cdot min^{-1}) = \dot{V}O_2\ (ml \cdot kg^{-1} \cdot min^{-1}) \times \text{body weight (kg)}$$
$$= (29.4\ ml \cdot kg^{-1} \cdot min^{-1}) \times (78.2\ kg)$$
$$= 2299\ ml \cdot min^{-1}$$

e) calculate resting component (Rest)

$$\text{Rest} = 3.5\ ml \cdot kg^{-1} \cdot min^{-1} \times kg\ \text{(body weight)}$$
$$= 3.5\ ml \cdot kg^{-1} \cdot min^{-1} \times 78.2\ kg$$
$$= 274\ ml \cdot min^{-1}$$

f) use leg ergometry formula to calculate the resistive component (RC)

$$\dot{V}O_2 = HC + RC + Rest$$
$$= O + RC + Rest$$
$$= RC + Rest$$

$$\therefore RC = \dot{V}O_2 - Rest$$
$$= 2299\ ml \cdot min^{-1} - 274\ ml \cdot min^{-1}$$
$$= 2025\ ml \cdot min^{-1}$$

g) calculate mechanical power (P) from RC

$$RC\ (ml \cdot min^{-1}) = P\ (kg \cdot m \cdot min^{-1}) \times 2\ (ml \cdot kg^{-1} \cdot m^{-1})$$

$$\therefore P = \frac{RC\ (ml \cdot min^{-1})}{2\ (ml \cdot kg^{-1} \cdot m^{-1})}$$
$$= \frac{2025\ ml \cdot min^{-1}}{2\ ml \cdot kg^{-1} \cdot m^{-1}}$$
$$= 1013\ kg \cdot m \cdot min^{-1}$$

Table D-1. Summary of Metabolic Calculations

$\dot{V}O_2$ Mode (units)	=	Horizontal Component	+	Vertical or Resistive Component	+	Resting Component	Comments
Walking $(ml \cdot kg^{-1} \cdot min^{-1})$	=	$m \cdot min^{-1} \times \left(0.1 \frac{ml \cdot kg^{-1} \cdot min^{-1}}{m \cdot min^{-1}}\right)$	+	grade (frac) $\times\ m \cdot min^{-1} \times 1.8 \frac{ml \cdot kg^{-1} \cdot min^{-1}}{m \cdot min^{-1}}$	+	$3.5\ ml \cdot kg^{-1} \cdot min^{-1}$	1. For speeds of 50–100 $m \cdot min^{-1}$ (1.9–3.7 $mi \cdot h^{-1}$) 2. $1.8 \frac{ml}{kg \cdot m} \times \frac{m \cdot min^{-1}}{m \cdot min^{-1}} = 1.8 \frac{ml \cdot kg^{-1} \cdot min^{-1}}{m \cdot min^{-1}}$ 3. $1\ mi \cdot h^{-1} = 26.8\ m \cdot min^{-1}$
Running $(ml \cdot kg^{-1} \cdot min^{-1})$	=	$m \cdot min^{-1} \times \left(0.2 \frac{ml \cdot kg^{-1} \cdot min^{-1}}{m \cdot min^{-1}}\right)$ ▲	+	grade (frac) $\times\ m \cdot min^{-1} \times 1.8 \frac{ml \cdot kg^{-1} \cdot min^{-1}}{m \cdot min^{-1}} \times 0.5$ ▲	+	$3.5\ ml \cdot kg^{-1} \cdot min^{-1}$	1. For speeds >134 $m \cdot min^{-1}$ (>5.0 $mi \cdot h^{-1}$) 2. If truly jogging (not walking), this equation can also be used for speeds between 80 and 134 $m \cdot min^{-1}$ (3–5 $mi \cdot h^{-1}$) 3. Formula applies to level running off the treadmill, but not to grade running off the treadmill
Leg Ergometer $(ml \cdot min^{-1})$	=	None	+	$\frac{kg \cdot m}{min} \times \frac{2\ ml}{kg \cdot m}$	+	$3.5\ ml \cdot kg^{-1} \cdot min^{-1} \times kg$ (BW)	1. For work rates between 300–1200 $kg \cdot m \cdot min^{-1}$ 2. $\frac{kg \cdot m}{min} = kg \times \frac{m}{rev} \times \frac{rev}{min}$

				▲		▲	3. Multiply resting component by body weight (kg) to convert to $ml \cdot min^{-1}$ 4. Monarch = 6 $m \cdot rev^{-1}$ Tunturi = 3 $m \cdot rev^{-1}$
▨ Arm Ergometer ($ml \cdot min^{-1}$)	=	None	+	▨ $\frac{kg \cdot m}{min} \times 3 \frac{ml}{kg \cdot m}$ ▲	+	3.5 $ml \cdot kg^{-1} \cdot min^{-1}$ × kg (BW) ▲	1. For work rates between 150–750 $kg \cdot m \cdot min^{-1}$ 2. $\frac{kg \cdot m}{min} = kg \times \frac{m}{rev} \times \frac{rev}{min}$ 3. Multiply resting component by body weight (kg) to convert to $ml \cdot min^{-1}$
▨ Stepping ($ml \cdot kg^{-1} \cdot min^{-1}$)	=	▨ $\frac{steps}{min} \times 0.35 \frac{ml \cdot kg^{-1} \cdot min^{-1}}{steps \cdot min^{-1}}$ ▲	+	▨ ▨ $\frac{m}{steps} \times \frac{steps}{min} \times 1.33$ $\times 1.8 \frac{ml \cdot kg^{-1} \cdot min^{-1}}{m \cdot min^{-1}}$	+	Included in horizontal and vertical components ▲	1. 1.33 includes both positive component of going up (1.0) + negative component of going down (0.33) = 1.33 2. Stepping height in meters.

Key: ▨ possible unknown quantity
▲ note change in constant

h) convert $kg \cdot m \cdot min^{-1}$ to watts, the appropriate SI unit

$$P\ (\text{watts}) = P\ (kg \cdot m \cdot min^{-1}) \times \left(\frac{1\ \text{watt}}{6\ kg \cdot m \cdot min^{-1}}\right)$$

$$= (1013\ \cancel{kg \cdot m \cdot min^{-1}}) \times \left(\frac{1\ \text{watt}}{6\ \cancel{kg \cdot m \cdot min^{-1}}}\right)$$

$$= 169\ \text{watts}$$

Example 3:

If the subject in example 2 desired to pedal at 80 rpm ($rev \cdot min^{-1}$) on an ergometer with a flywheel that travels 6 $m \cdot rev^{-1}$, how much weight or load should be placed on the ergometer?

a) calculate weight or force (F) applied in kg

$$P\ (kg \cdot m \cdot min^{-1}) = F\ (kg) \times (m \cdot rev^{-1}) \times (rev \cdot min^{-1})$$

$$\therefore F\ (kg) = \frac{P\ (kg \cdot m \cdot min^{-1})}{(m \cdot rev^{-1}) \times (rev \cdot min^{-1})}$$

$$= \frac{1013\ kg \cdot \cancel{m} \cdot \cancel{min^{-1}}}{(6\ \cancel{m} \cdot \cancel{rev^{-1}}) \times (80\ \cancel{rev} \cdot \cancel{min^{-1}})}$$

$$= 2.1\ kg$$

Table D–2. Approximate Energy Requirements in METs For Horizontal and Grade Walking

% Grade	$mi \cdot h^{-1}$	1.7	2.0	2.5	3.0	3.4	3.75
	$m \cdot min^{-1}$	45.6	53.7	67.0	80.5	91.2	100.5
0		2.3	2.5	2.9	3.3	3.6	3.9
2.5		2.9	3.2	3.8	4.3	4.8	5.2
5.0		3.5	3.9	4.6	5.4	5.9	6.5
7.5		4.1	4.6	5.5	6.4	7.1	7.8
10.0		4.6	5.3	6.3	7.4	8.3	9.1
12.5		5.2	6.0	7.2	8.5	9.5	10.4
15.0		5.8	6.6	8.1	9.5	10.6	11.7
17.5		6.4	7.3	8.9	10.5	11.8	12.9
20.0		7.0	8.0	9.8	11.6	13.0	14.2
22.5		7.6	8.7	10.6	12.6	14.2	15.5
25.0		8.2	9.4	11.5	13.6	15.3	16.8

Table D-3. Approximate Energy Requirements in METS for Horizontal and Uphill Jogging/Running

a. Outdoors on solid surface

% Grade	$m \cdot h^{-1}$	5	6	7	7.5	8	9	10
	$m \cdot min^{-1}$	134	161	188	201	215	241	268
0		8.6	10.2	11.7	12.5	13.3	14.8	16.3
2.5		10.3	12.3	14.1	15.1	16.1	17.9	19.7
5.0		12.0	14.3	16.5	17.7	18.8		
7.5		13.8	16.4	18.9				
10.0		15.5	18.5					

b. On the treadmill

% Grade	$m \cdot h^{-1}$	5	6	7	7.5	8	9	10
	$m \cdot min^{-1}$	134	161	188	201	215	241	268
0		8.6	10.2	11.7	12.5	13.3	14.8	16.3
2.5		9.5	11.2	12.9	13.8	14.7	16.3	18.0
5.0		10.3	12.3	14.1	15.1	16.1	17.9	19.7
7.5		11.2	13.3	15.3	16.4	17.4	19.4	
10.0		12.0	14.3	16.5	17.7	18.8		
12.5		12.9	15.4	17.7	19.0			
15.0		13.8	16.4	18.9				

Table D–4. Approximate Energy Expenditure in METs During Bicycle Ergometry

Body Weight		Exercise Rate (kg·m·min⁻¹ and Watts)						
kg	lb	300 / 50	450 / 75	600 / 100	750 / 125	900 / 150	1050 / 175	1200 ($kg \cdot m \cdot min^{-1}$), 200 (Watts)
50	110	5.1	6.9	8.6	10.3	12.0	13.7	15.4
60	132	4.3	5.7	7.1	8.6	10.0	11.4	12.9
70	154	3.7	4.9	6.1	7.3	8.6	9.8	11.0
80	176	3.2	4.3	5.4	6.4	7.5	8.6	9.6
90	198	2.9	3.8	4.8	5.7	6.7	7.6	8.6
100	220	2.6	3.4	4.3	5.1	6.0	6.9	7.7

NOTE: $\dot{V}O_2$ for zero load pedaling is approximately 550 $ml \cdot min^{-1}$ for 70 to 80 kg subjects.

SELECTED REFERENCES

Adams, WC: Influence of age, sex and body weight on the energy expenditure of bicycle riding. *J. Appl. Physiol. 22*:539–545, 1967.

Astrand, PO: Work tests with the bicycle ergometer. Varberg, Sweden: Monark-Crescent AB, (undated).

Claremont, A, Reddan WG, Smith, EL: Metabolic costs and feasibility of water support exercises for the elderly. In: Nagle FJ, Montoye HJ, (eds). *Exercise in Health and Disease.* Springfield: Charles C Thomas, 1981, pp. 215–225.

Dill, DB: Oxygen used in horizontal and grade walking and running on the treadmill. *J. Appl. Physiol. 20*:19–22, 1965.

Franklin BA, Vander L, Wrisley D, Rubenfire M: Aerobic requirements of arm ergometry: implications for exercise testing and training. *Phys. Spts. Med. 11*:81–90, 1983.

Katch VL, Villanacci JF, and Sady, SP: Energy costs of rebound-running. *Res. Quart. Exer. Spt. 52*:269–272, 1981.

Knuttgen, HG: Force, work, power and exercise. *Med. Sci. Spts. 10*:227–228, 1978.

Legwold G: Does aerobic dance offer more fun than fitness? *Phys. Spts. Med. 10*:147–151, 1982.

Magaria R, et al: Energy cost of running. *J. Appl. Physiol. 18*:367–370, 1963.

Nagle FJ, Balke B, and Naughton JP: Gradational step tests for assessing work capacity. *J. Appl. Physiol. 20*:745–748, 1965.

Nagle FJ, et al: Compatibility of progressive treadmill, bicycle and step tests based on oxygen uptake responses. *Med. Sci. Spts. 3*:149–154, 1971.

Passmore R, Durnin JVGA: Human energy expenditure. *Physiol. Rev. 35*:801–840, 1955.

INDEX

Page numbers in *italics* indicate illustrations; those followed by "t" indicate tables.